HANDBOOK OF VETERINARY NURSING

HANDBOOK OF
VETERINARY
NURSING

Hilary Orpet

and

Perdi Welsh

**Blackwell
Science**

DISTRIBUTORS
Marston Book Services Ltd
PO Box 269
Abingdon
Oxon OX14 4YN
(*Orders:* Tel: 01235 465500
     Fax: 01235 465555

USA and Canada
 Iowa State University Press
 A Blackwell Science Company
 2121 S. State Avenue
 Ames, Iowa 50014-8300
 (*Orders:* Tel: 800-862-6657
      Fax: 515-292-3348
      Web   www.isupress.com
      email: orders@isupress.com

Australia
 Blackwell Science Pty Ltd
 54 University Street
 Carlton, Victoria 3053
 (*Orders:* Tel: 03 9347 0300
      Fax: 03 9347 5001)

A catalogue record for this title
is available from the British Library

ISBN 0-632-05258-9

Library of Congress
Cataloging-in-Publication Data
Orpet. H. (Hilary)
 Handbook of veterinary nursing/by H. Orpet
 and P. Welsh.
    p. cm.
 Includes bibliographical references (p.).
 ISBN 0-632-05258-9
 1. Veterinary nursing – Handbooks, manuals,
 etc.   I. Welsh, P. (Perdi)   II. Title.

 SF774.5 .O77 2001
 636.089′073–dc21
                                        2001043327

For further information on
Blackwell Science, visit our website:
www.blackwell-science.com

CONTENTS

PREFACE

The aim of this book is to provide the veterinary nurse with a quick reference point for many of the nursing procedures he or she may come across in the clinical situation.

It is a resource for veterinary nurses at all stages of their training and levels of experience. For those at the beginning of their training and performing tasks for the first time, it gives clear and concise written instruction and diagrams. It should be of particular benefit to those nurses who are studying and preparing for their Royal College of Veterinary Surgeons (RCVS) Level Three Oral and Practical examinations as the practical skills are set out in a clear step-by-step format. For those veterinary nurses with many years of experience it may be used as a reminder and quick reference source for some of the more advanced nursing skills such as jugular catheter placement and skin suture patterns.

The format is designed to provide the reader with easy access to clinical procedures, calculations and care plans, all of which have been written in bullet points. It is not intended that this handbook is taken as an absolute, but used as a guide for practices to devise their own work plans to ensure that all aspects of nursing are considered and acted upon to the highest of standards.

The book highlights the importance of working methodically, to a systematic routine and by standardising procedures will help to ensure that the whole team work to certain formats which in turn will help to ensure the most successful outcomes.

As this is primarily about *clinical skills procedures* it is not within the scope of the book to provide underpinning knowledge for each topic but the reader may make use of the references at the end of each chapter for further information on each subject.

The book is intended to be a guide to quality care and skills, however, none of the procedures should be carried out without appropriate instruction first and then only under the direction of a veterinary surgeon. Veterinary nurses must be familiar with and work within the RCVS *Guide to Professional Conduct* and keep up to date with the ongoing amendments and reviews to The Veterinary Surgeons Act 1966 Schedule 3 which allows nonvets to undertake certain acts of veterinary surgery.

The authors have been involved in veterinary nurse training and education for many years. Both have worked at the university teaching hospital at the Royal Veterinary College as well as in private practice. They are examiners for the RCVS Oral and Practical examinations. With these combined skills and knowledge they have collaborated to write a book for veterinary nurses who wish to develop and provide quality nursing care.

Hilary Orpet
VN DipAVN (Surgical) CertEd

Perdi Welsh
VN DipAVN (Surgical) CertEd

SECTION 1
THE WARD

CHAPTER 1

WARD MANAGEMENT – INTRODUCTION

The task of nursing animals through disease or debilitation is taken on by the Veterinary Nurse (VN). The skills of the VN play an essential role in speeding up recovery times and generally making the patient feel more comfortable during any stay. The VN must be able to carry out many procedures confidently and be able to recognise normal and abnormal clinical signs and symptoms.

Veterinary nurses are involved in:

- Observation
- Management
- Care

of *every* patient.

A daily schedule that is adhered to will reduce the risk of important points being overlooked during busy days and ensure more efficient and effective care of the patient. Protocols can be established as a helpful reminder of all of the different aspects of the patient's care and help maintain a high standard of management.

ITEMS TO BE INCLUDED ON A DAILY SCHEDULE

COMMUNICATION

Essential between the Veterinary Surgeon (VS) and Veterinary Nurse (VN) with regard to each patient. Initial information given on admittance and then at least twice daily after that. A regular update on the animal's state of health and demeanour will identify special needs and enable changes in treatment or management to be discussed.

RECORD-KEEPING

Thorough and accurate records are essential. Changes can only be properly identified when they are written down and compared with previous recordings. It also enables other members of the practice to become familiar with the case by perusal of the record sheet. See Fig. 1.1.

Case Number		Medication	
Clinical summary			

Date	Day number			Date	Day number			
Weight				Weight				
Temp.				Temp.				
Pulse				Pulse				
Resp.				Resp.				
Food				Food				
Liquid				Liquid				
Urine				Urine				
Faeces				Faeces				
MEDICATION				MEDICATION				
PROCEDURE				PROCEDURE				
COMMENTS				COMMENTS				

Fig. 1.1 Example of a case record sheet.

PHYSICAL EXAMINATION

At least once a day, the VN should carry out a full physical examination of each patient. Abnormalities can then be identified early and treated appropriately. Temperature, pulse and respiration monitoring should be standard procedure for every animal. Further information regarding appetite, urination, defecation, vomiting, diarrhoea and any other abnormalities should be observed and recorded. Animals recovering from anaesthesia should have particular attention paid to monitoring of vital signs until fully recovered.

EXERCISE AND TOILETING

The VN must ensure that all animals are given the chance to urinate and defecate in a way that is most comfortable for them. For example, cats need clean litter trays and some may desire more privacy (place litter tray inside a box). Some dogs will only urinate on grass whilst others will urinate only on concrete. Try to identify what they are happiest with and ask owners if necessary. Take out as often as appropriate for each animal. (Polydipsic patients and animals receiving diuretic treatment will require more frequent opportunities to urinate). The type and amount of exercise will depend on the animal's condition. Particular care must be taken with postsurgical cases, cardiac and respiratory cases. Discuss exercise management with the VS.

WOUND CARE

All surgical wounds must be examined daily for evidence of haemorrhage, inflammation, infection or patient interference. Understand the principles of wound healing and management to ensure the best possible outcome for wound healing. Keep up to date with new dressing materials and select the most appropriate for each wound at each stage of its healing.

PHYSIOTHERAPY

Physiotherapy is grossly under-utilised in veterinary practice. It can dramatically improve the physical and mental well-being of the patient and may speed up the rehabilitation process. Massage, active exercise and hydrotherapy are inexpensive and with a little basic training can be performed by the VN.

FLUID THERAPY

The VN must have practical knowledge of catheter placement, aseptic management of administration lines, calculation of fluid deficits and maintenance rates, and the monitoring of the animal during administration.

SPECIAL DIETS AND NUTRITION

Many patients are physically unable to eat, and others become inappetent due to the stress of hospitalisation or illness. Injured and diseased animals have an increased metabolic rate and will become severely nutritionally compromised after only a few days without food. Anorexic patients must be identified quickly so that appropriate action can be taken. Nutritional support may be administered by assisted oral feeding, nasogastric feeding or gastrostomy tube. The calculation of daily calorie requirement based on basal energy requirements (BER) should be worked out and feeding tubes managed correctly. Patients with specific diseases may require prescription foods or different life stage foods and postoperative diets should be given appropriately. Observation of water intake and availability is essential.

ADMINISTRATION OF MEDICINES

The VN must be confident in administration of medicines as prescribed by the VS. Correct calculation of drug doses is essential. Administration of the incorrect dose of many drugs can kill patients! *Learn how to calculate drug dosages accurately.* Adhere to prescribed treatment times.

PATIENT CLEANING AND GROOMING

Cleaning the animal, removing discharges from eyes, nose, mouth, etc., will help it feel much better. It is also a useful method of improving the nurse/patient relationship and will help to speed the animal's overall recovery. Many hospitalised animals will not groom themselves either because of debilitation or stress. Grooming is required not only to remove excess hair but also to help identify skin lesions or parasites. In addition, grooming improves the patient's demeanour and helps show the owner that care and attention is being paid to their pet.

WARD HYGIENE

It is the VN's role to ensure effective disinfection of kennels and equipment to prevent cross-infection and nosocomial infections. Patients suspected of, or known to have a contagious/zoonotic disease should be isolated. Restricted access to these cases should reduce the risk of spread to other patients and staff. Personal hygiene must be carried out before handling each patient, their fluid administration lines, wounds and before giving any injections, etc. All faeces, urine, vomit, etc., must be cleaned immediately and food must not be left around for too long as it will go off and attract flies.

RUNNING AN ISOLATION UNIT

Any animal that is suspected of having an infectious disease should be admitted into the isolation unit, away from any other animal. They should have their own outside runs, bedding and bowls. Personnel should wear specific clothing and carry out scrupulous hygiene procedures after handling any infectious animal. This is called *barrier* or *isolation nursing*.

Remember that infectious diseases can be transmitted by:

- *Direct contact*: animal is in close contact with another or bites from fights
- *Indirect contact*: aerosol droplets, people, inanimate objects, e.g. food bowls, bedding and kennels

BASIC DESIGN OF THE ISOLATION UNIT

The isolation unit should be a totally self-contained unit, containing all the bedding, feeding, monitoring and fluid therapy equipment required by each particular case.

As with all kennelling, there should be an active ventilation system, which allows 6–12 air changes per hour. Heating systems must be thermostatically controlled to provide the required ambient temperature for each animal, bearing in mind that many isolated cases have the potential to become hypo-

THE WARD

THE WARD

thermic easily. This is of particular importance to animals with severe diarrhoea, for whom provision of blankets can be difficult.

The walls and floors should be easy to clean and disinfect, ideally with a central drainage system to enable the whole room to be hosed down and disinfected.

There should be as little clutter as possible. Keep all equipment and bedding, etc., in closed cupboards and keep surfaces clear. Remember that inanimate objects can transmit disease.

Written protocols can help to ensure that barrier nursing is carried out effectively by everyone:

ISOLATION UNIT PROTOCOL

(1) Keep the patient's records and hospitalisation sheet on the outside of the room so that anyone can peruse them without having to enter the room.

(2) Place a sign on the front of the door to the unit to warn staff what the potential danger is, e.g. canine parvovirus, leptospirosis, etc.

(3) Wear shoe covers or specific footwear, and disposable gowns, gloves and mask when handling the patient or cleaning the kennel.

(4) Dispose of protective clothing into the clinical waste bins.

(5) Wash hands thoroughly in an antiseptic solution upon leaving the unit.

(6) Place a foot-bath (litter tray filled with disinfectant solution) just outside the door of the unit and instruct personnel to walk through it when leaving the isolation unit.

(7) Involve as few people as possible in the treatment of the patient (i.e. the attending veterinary surgeon and one nurse).

(8) Attend to the patient *after* treating any other inpatients and not *before* treating them. Isolation staff are not subsequently to attend to young or old animals or those who are immunosuppressed.

(9) Provide the patient with disposable bedding such as newspaper and incontinence sheets. Dispose of all bedding into clinical waste bins.

(10) Wash all used food bowls in detergent, and leave to soak in a disinfectant solution for appropriate length of time. Autoclave metal bowls before using for another animal.

(11) Do not allow the patient to come into contact with any other animal during its stay.
(12) Take isolated patient to a separate designated run or area, to urinate and defecate.
(13) Clear away all urine, faeces, vomit, etc., as soon as it is voided and use disinfectant as recommended by the manufacturers.

OTHER CONSIDERATIONS

- All hospitalised animals should be kept warm in draught-free kennels. Very young or very old animals are unable to conserve their body heat and so become cold easily.
- Some animals (reptiles) are *poikilothermic*, i.e. their body temperature depends on ambient temperature.
- Remember that recumbent animals are unable to move away from heat sources and may become burnt.
- Make sure animals do not chew electrical flexes.

It is important to ensure that all hospitalised animals are comfortable. Recumbent animals require additional foam padding to prevent bedsores and should be turned when necessary. Small animals such as rabbits and wildlife may be terrified in the hospital environment and may need boxes and hay to hide in.

Mental stimulation is often important to help speed recovery, improve mental attitude and help prevent boredom. Recumbent patients in particular need a lot of attention. Toys for cats can be made out of old syringe cases and dog chews given to dogs. Blankets and toys from home sometimes help.

THE WARD

CHAPTER 2

CLEANING AND DISINFECTION OF ANIMAL ACCOMMODATION

Good hygiene and effective disinfection of animal accommodation, associated equipment and personal hygiene is essential to help prevent the spread of *communicable* diseases and *nosocomial* infections.

The most usual means of spreading infection include:

- Hands of staff involved
- Inanimate objects (bedding, kennels, brushes, food bowls, etc.)
- Dust particles or droplet nuclei suspended in the atmosphere

The VN is responsible for ensuring that spread of infection is minimised and therefore must know how to clean, what to clean and what to use.

SELECTING THE APPROPRIATE PRODUCT

DETERGENTS

Detergents are primarily soap cleansing agents such as washing up liquid and washing powder. They do not necessarily destroy micro-organisms although transient bacteria may almost be removed by thorough washing with such an agent and water. The main function of detergents in practice is to remove dirt, grease, body fluids and other organic materials in preparation for *disinfection* or *sterilisation*.

DISINFECTANTS

Disinfectants remove or destroy micro-organisms (although not always bacterial spores) in the environment. They must be used in accordance with the manufacturer's recommendations to ensure their effectiveness.

ANTISEPTICS

Antiseptics remove or destroy micro-organisms on the skin.

The following should be taken into consideration when selecting a particular antiseptic or disinfectant:

- Effectiveness against particular organisms, e.g. parvovirus
- Effectiveness against a wide range of micro-organisms (gram-negative bacteria and bacterial spores, fungi and viruses which are more resistant than gram-positive bacteria)
- Toxic and irritant effects to operators and animals
- Effectiveness in the presence of a wide range or organic and inorganic materials
- Stability of product in storage or once made up
- Smell of the product
- Cost of the product
- Staining or corrosive effects on certain materials
- Contact time required
- Ease of use
- Control of Substances Hazardous to Health (COSHH) regulations 1999 and handling precautions required
- Effectiveness in different temperatures of water
- Possible toxic or noxious effects when mixed with other substances such as detergents

CLEANING ACCOMMODATION AND EQUIPMENT

The protocol in Table 2.1 should be employed:

Equipment
Equipment must also be cleaned and disinfected regularly to maintain effective hospital hygiene. Types of disinfectant are shown in Table 2.2. Steps 3 to 9 listed in Table 2.1 may be utilised for general cleaning and disinfection of pieces of equipment shown below. In addition, some of these items may then require sterilisation using an appropriate method.

- Food bowls
- Grooming brushes
- Mops
- Shovels
- Bedding
- Bins
- Kitchen utensils

THE WARD

Table 2.1   Protocol for effective cleaning.

Action	Rationale
(1) Remove animal to secure outside run or temporary cage (must not be another animal's kennel)	Kennel cannot be cleaned effectively with animal inside and increases risk of escape
(2) Remove bedding, newspaper, food bowls and toys	Bedding and bowls for washing, dispose of other bedding materials appropriately
(3) Remove gross soiling (faeces, etc.) with shovel or dustpan	Dispose of appropriately
(4) Clean with detergent solution	To clean away dirt and debris to prepare for effective disinfection – many disinfectants are inactivated by organic matter
(5) Rinse with water to remove detergent	Many disinfectants produce noxious gases when mixed with detergent or become inactivated by these solutions
(6) Apply appropriate disinfectant taking into consideration their recommended use and dilution rates	Some species of animal are sensitive to some types of disinfectant (e.g. cats and phenol)
(7) Leave for recommended contact time	To ensure most effective destruction of pathogenic micro-organisms
(8) Rinse thoroughly	Strong odours may be offensive and/or irritant to some animals
(9) Dry thoroughly	To prevent animal's paws from becoming wet
(10) Replace fresh bedding materials if necessary	Prepare for next occupant
(11) Return animal to kennel if necessary	Secure animal

Points to remember when using disinfectants

- New products come onto the market all the time – keep up to date with new products and chemical compounds.
- Veterinary nurses must *always* look after their own safety and hygiene – wear appropriate protective clothing. This ranges from basic gloves and apron for all disinfectant products to wearing protective goggles and mask with others (aldehydes). Do not be lazy about this – effects may not be immediate but become evident years later.
- *Always* look after the safety of the patients – do not use chemicals that are irritant or toxic to them.
- Store disinfectants according to manufacturer's instructions and once made up use within recommended time.

Table 2.2 Types of disinfectant.

Groups of disinfectants	Other name/ chemical composition	Example of trade name	Qualities
Phenolics/phenols	Black fluids	Jeyes™ Fluid	Inexpensive Not easily inactivated Not very effective against viruses Toxic and irritant on skin Toxic to cats Strong-smelling Leaves sticky residue
	White fluids	Izal™	As above
	Clear fluids	Clearsol™	As above
	Chlorinated phenols – chloroxylenols	Dettol™, Ibcol™	Less irritant than above Easily inactivated by hard water and organic material
Halogen	Hypochlorite – bleach	Domestos™ Chloros™	Inexpensive Effective against wide range of bacteria and viruses, spores and fungi Strong smell Corrosive to metal Bleaches materials Gases released when mixed with acids (e.g. urine and some other cleaning agents) Inactivated by organic matter

Groups of disinfectants	Other name/ chemical composition	Example of trade name	Qualities
Halogenated tertiary amines (HTA)	Quarternary Ammonium Compounds (QACs)	Trigene™	Wide range of activity against bacteria, viruses, spores and fungi Not easily inactivated by organic material Low toxicity (gloves recommended) Noncorrosive Relatively expensive
Iodine/iodophors	Povidone-iodine	Pevidene™	Wide range of activity Staining occurs so not usually used in the environment – more commonly used as antiseptic solution
Peroxides	Hydrogen peroxide		Wide range of activity Fast acting Ineffective with organic matter Low irritation and toxicity
	Peroxygen compound	Virkon™	Fast-acting Active against wide range of organisms Available as a powder which is irritant until made up Not affected by organic matter Causes metal corrosion

Paracetic acid		Oxykill™, Vetcide 2000™	Fast-acting Highly irritant Effective against wide range of organisms Not easily inactivated Corrosive Strong smell
Alcohol	Isopropyl alcohol 70% Ethanol 70%	Surgical spirit Methylated spirit	Effective against bacteria but not spores and some viruses Inactivated by organic material Highly flammable Expensive Skin irritant
Aldehyde	Gluteraldehyde Formaldehyde (not used – too irritant)	Cidex™ Formula-H™ Gigasept™ Parvocide™ Vetcide™	Effective against a wide range of bacteria, spores and viruses Not inactivated easily Slow acting Highly toxic – causing skin and eye sensitivity and respiratory problems Activity is related to temperature Not recommended for general every day use
Dichloroisocyanurates	Sodium dichloro-isocyanurate NaDCC	Presept™ Vetaclean-Parvo™	Wide range of activity Not easily inactivated Irritant Highly corrosive to metals and textiles

CONTROL OF SUBSTANCES HAZARDOUS TO HEALTH REGULATIONS (COSHH) 1999

The COSSH regulations require that veterinary practices assess the potential risks associated with a disinfectant and then prevent or control exposure to staff. This information can be obtained from the safety data sheets associated with every product and gives details of maximum exposure limits (MEL) and occupational exposure standards (OES) for each product. A *standard operating procedure* (SOP) should be drawn up by every practice.

PERSONAL HYGIENE – ANTISEPTICS

Research in human nursing has shown that hand washing is the single most important procedure for preventing nosocomial infection as hands have been shown to be an important route of infection. Even wearing rings increases the number of micro-organisms on the hands. This research also showed that hand washing is rarely carried out in a satisfactory manner!

Antiseptics are used primarily to destroy or inhibit the growth of micro-organisms on the skin and mucous membranes. Many antiseptic solutions also contain a soap/detergent (surfactant) solution.

There are three main groups: chlorhexidine, iodine and alcohol (see *surgical scrub procedure* in Chapter 13).

CHAPTER 3

THE CLINICAL EXAMINATION OF SMALL ANIMALS

The clinical examination of the patient provides essential information about the state of health. A routine, systematic method of examination is required to detect abnormalities and this involves practice and thoroughness. Record *all* findings, normal as well as abnormal.

Before attempting a physical examination it is important to be able to handle and restrain the animal correctly.

APPROACHING THE ANIMAL

1 Observe behaviour and assess the animal, ask the owner
2 Approach quietly and confidently – using its name and talking in a reassuring manner
3 Bend down to the animal's level
4 Offer closed fist for the animal to sniff if no signs of aggression are seen

Remember:

- Animals often behave better away from the owners
- When taking a dog from an owner, take the owner and dog into a room away from the waiting room
- Use a slip lead as dogs may often slip their collars
- Ask the owner to leave the room rather than dragging the dog from the room

CAUSES OF AGGRESSION IN ANIMALS

- Dominance
- Possessiveness – territorial, food, owner
- Fear
- Pain

- Maternal protection
- Breed predisposition (such as guard dogs and working dogs)
- Too much restraint! (especially in brachycephalic dogs)

MOVING ANIMALS AROUND THE PRACTICE

CATS

Cats should *always* be transported around the practice securely in a basket. A cat that is carried in the arms may easily be frightened and escape!

Equipment for controlling aggressive cats
There are various pieces of equipment that can be used to control an aggressive cat. Make sure you know how to use them correctly.

- Cat catcher
- Thick towel
- Mikki muzzle
- Crush cage
- Leather gauntlets
- Cat bag

DOGS

When taking a dog from one area to another ensure it has a secure lead attached. Slip leads are routinely used as the dog cannot easily 'back' out of it!

Carrying and lifting
Many VNs suffer from back problems from lifting incorrectly. Attempting to lift a dog that is too heavy may result in injury to the VN and the dog. Animals often struggle if they do not feel secure when they are being carried. Always ensure that there is adequate control over an animal so that no one gets injured.

When lifting large dogs (greater than 25 kg), two or more people are required. Always ensure the dog's head is controlled and that the animal is well supported. For smaller dogs it is sufficient to ensure the dog's head is controlled and the body is well supported.

Equipment for controlling aggressive dogs

- Dog catcher
- Muzzle
- Mikki
- Baskerville
- Bandage tape muzzle

Whether handling an aggressive cat or dog, remember

- Be firm
- Be confident
- Be positive

SMALL MAMMALS

Small mammals are often transported in cat carriers. Make sure they cannot escape through the wire mesh or air holes. Rodents are best *not* transported in cardboard boxes, as they will often eat their way out. See Table 3.1 for handling small animals.

Table 3.1   Handling and restraint of small animals.

Animal	Method of restraint
Rabbits	Handle carefully and quietly
	Scruff if necessary and support the hind quarters
	If frightened or handled roughly, rabbits can easily damage their spine and become paralysed
	Do not pick up by their ears
Guinea-pigs	Place one hand around the shoulders and support the hindquarters
	Most guinea-pigs are reasonably tame – but do not frighten or startle
Rats	Rats rarely bite unless frightened or in pain
	Pick up by placing a hand around the shoulders
	Position the thumb under the mandible to prevent biting
	Scruffing rats causes considerable distress
Mice	Mice may bite if frightened – handle with care
	Scruff gently and grip base of tail with 3rd or 4th finger
Gerbils	Pick up by gently cupping hands around the animal
	Restrain by holding *base* of tail If more restraint is required – gently hold by the scruff
	Take care that it doesn't jump off the table
Hamsters	Handle with care!
	Hamsters can inflict painful bites
	Pick up by gently cupping hands around the animal
	Further restraint may be by 'scruffing' gently
Budgerigar	Hold head gently between 1st and 2nd finger
	Take care not to asphyxiate bird!

THE WARD

BIRDS

Birds are often brought to the surgery in their own cages. Make sure they are placed in a quiet, darkened area to keep them calm and reduce stress. Birds that arrive in small cardboard boxes are fine for a short period only – they should ideally be transferred to a larger cage.

CLINICAL EXAMINATION – VISUAL INSPECTION AND OBSERVATION

PROCEDURE

(1) Observe the patient from a distance. Apprehension, fear or excitement is normal in a strange environment. However, look to see if the patient appears depressed, lethargic or distressed.
(2) Look at the overall condition of the coat and note any hair loss, scaling, pustules, injuries, parasites and wounds.
(3) Check whether the animal appears emaciated or obese and observe for any apparent lameness, weakness or neurological defects.
(4) Before handling the patient, watch the respiration rate and depth.
(5) Approach the animal for a closer examination. Do this slowly and talk to the patient whilst doing so.

Gaining the animal's confidence will enable an easier and more accurate evaluation. Figure 3.1 shows the measurement of vital signs.

VITAL SIGNS – TEMPERATURE, PULSE AND RESPIRATION

1. Taking a rectal temperature
A rectal temperature should be obtained. This is sometimes best left until the end of the examination so as not to stress the animal too much. See Table 3.2 for normal ranges.

Procedure

(1) *Restrain* patient adequately
(2) *Shake* the thermometer (to ensure the mercury returns to the bulb)

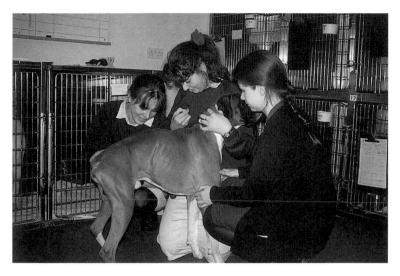

Fig. 3.1 Measuring vital signs.

THE WARD

(3) *Lubricate* with Vaseline, KY jelly or similar
(4) *Insert* gently into the rectum and hold thermometer tip against rectal wall
(5) *Time* for at least 30 seconds
(6) *Read* and *record* temperature
(7) *Clean* thermometer: wipe excess faecal matter, clean and disinfect. Leave in appropriate place (disinfectant thermometer stand or plastic casing)

Table 3.2 Normal ranges for rectal temperature.

Species	Temperature in °C	Temperature in °F
Dog	38.3–38.7	100.9–101.7
Cat	38.0–38.5	100.4–101.6
Neonatal dogs and cats	35.5–36.1	96.0–97.0
Rabbit	37.0–39.4	99.0–103.0
Guinea-pig	39.0–40.0	102.2–104.2
Hamster	36.0–38.0	98.0–101.0
Gerbil	38.0–39.0	100.4–102.2
Ferret	37.8–40.0	100.4–104.2
Chinchilla	38.0–39.0	100.4–102.2
Rat	37.5–38.0	99.8–100.5

2. Recording the pulse rate
A pulse can be felt by light palpation of an artery. Each pulsation corresponds to the contraction of the *left ventricle* of the heart and is usually assessed at the same time as listening

Table 3.3 Normal pulse rates.

Species	Normal heart rate per minute
Dog	60–120
Neonatal dogs and cats	200–220
Cat	100–140
Rabbit	205–235
Guinea pig	130–190
Hamster	300–600
Gerbil	100–150
Ferret	300–400
Chinchilla	100–150
Rat	260–340

to the heart. See Table 3.3 for normal ranges. The pulse rate may increase with each inspiration and decrease on expiration. This is called sinus arrythmia and is considered to be a normal variation.

A pulse may be felt at various sites where the artery runs close to the body surface.

- Femoral: inner thigh
- Digital: palmar aspect of carpus
- Tarsal: medial surface of tarsus
- Coccygeal: ventral aspect of tail base
- Sublingual: under the tongue (in anaesthetised patients)

Procedure

(1) Restrain the animal
(2) Locate pulse
(3) Count pulsations over one minute
(4) Record the rate and report abnormalities
(5) Check the pulse rate with the heart rate to check for pulse deficits

3. Recording respiration rate

Ideally respiration should be noted with the animal at rest *before* exciting it with an examination. See Table 3.4 for normal ranges.

Table 3.4 Normal respiration rates.

Species	Normal respiration rate per minute
Dog	15–30
Cat	20–30
Neonatal dogs and cats	15–35
Rabbit	38–65
Guinea-pig	90–150
Hamster	33–127
Gerbil	40–80
Ferret	30–40
Chinchilla	40–80
Rat	70–150

Procedure
Either

(1) Gently place the hands either side of the chest cavity and count the number of respirations by feeling the movement of the chest

or,

(2) Carefully observe the movement of the chest wall while the animal is resting, counting the number of respirations over one minute

The depth should also be noted.

HEAD TO TAIL EXAMINATION

1. Head

Examine the eyes, ears, nose and mouth for evidence of discharge, changes in size and shape.

Eyes

Inspect the eye and external orbital structures. The eyelids should touch the globe, but the eyelashes should not touch the surface of the cornea. Examine the conjunctiva and sclera for evidence of infection, exudates and petechia and check their colour. Check the pupillary light reflex.

Mouth

Gently retract the lips and examine the teeth and gums. Smell the breath, and take note of any discharges or excess saliva. Examine the mucous membranes. The capillary refill time (CRT) should be less than 2 seconds. Slow CRTs indicate that peripheral perfusion is poor, this may be due to dehydration or shock. The colour of the mucous membranes should be pink. Bright red membranes may indicate septic shock or carbon monoxide poisoning, pale membranes indicate anaemia, hypovolaemia and blue membranes may indicate inadequate oxygenation. Examine the teeth for staining, faulty enamel, calculus, caries and loose or broken teeth. Check the dentition and note whether permanent or deciduous teeth are present. Dental formulae for dogs and cats are shown in Table 3.5.

2. Lymph nodes
Superficial palpable lymph nodes:

- Submandibular
- Prescapular
- Axillary
- Popliteal
- Inguinal

These lymph nodes should be palpated to identify enlargement indicating inflammatory, infectious or neoplastic conditions.

3. Thorax
Auscultate the thorax using a stethoscope to assess the presence of pulmonary or cardiac problems.

Listen to the heart first. Make a note of the rate and rhythm of the heartbeat. Listen for murmurs of abnormal sounds. The normal heart sound is described to sound like 'lub-dub'. Inform the veterinary surgeon if the heart sounds are muffled. This may indicate pleural effusion, intrathoracic masses or diaphragmatic hernias. Take a femoral pulse whilst listening to the heart to confirm synchronicity. If the heart rate is higher than the pulse rate it indicates that a pulse deficit exists. Then listen to the lungs by moving the stethoscope from the dorsal thorax down to the ventral thorax. Usually soft blowing

Table 3.5   Dental formulae for the dog and cat.

	Dental formulae			
Deciduous dentition in the dog	incisors 3/3	canines 1/1	molars 3/2	
Permanent dentition in the dog	Incisors 3/3	Canines 1/1	Premolars 4/4	Molars 2/3
Deciduous dentition in the cat	incisors 3/3	canines 1/1	molars 3/2	
Permanent dentition in the cat	Incisors 3/3	Canines 1/1	Premolars 3/2	Molars 1/1

sounds are heard. Abnormal sounds such as crackles, wheezes, pops or squeaks should be noted.

4. Abdomen

Abdominal palpation requires skill and practice. It can potentially cause harm if carried out by the inexperienced. As a guide, the animal should be positioned on the examination table, with its head facing away from you. Without touching the animal, inspect the abdomen for general contour, presence of swelling and generalised distension. Observe the movement of the abdominal walls during respiration. Check that the animal is standing freely rather than 'tucked-up' or hunched.

5. Genitalia and perineal region

In the male, examine the prepuce and anus for evidence of discharge or haemorrhage. Palpate the testes to ensure symmetry. Palpate and examine the vulva and mammary glands in the female. In cases of paralysis, the anal sphincter reflex can be examined.

6. Limbs

Examine the lymph nodes surrounding the fore and hind limbs. Inspect and palpate the legs and joints, looking for pain, heat, swelling, deformities and restricted movement.

7. Weight

An accurate body weight for each animal should be obtained every day. Also visually assess to detect overall changes – emaciation or obesity. Losses of more than 10% of initial weight may require supportive nutrition and fluid therapy. (e.g. 10 kg dog losing 1 kg or 20 kg dog losing 2 kg of weight).

THE WARD

CHAPTER 4

NUTRITIONAL SUPPORT

The VN plays an important role in feeding of patients; firstly he or she needs to be aware of when certain patients may require encouragement to feed or need to be tube fed; and report to the VS in charge of the case.

The VN should then help to decide on an appropriate feeding regime to suit the needs of each patient's temperament and physical condition, maintain the feeding equipment and tubes in use and calculate the daily calorie requirements according to the patient's disease or condition.

Patients requiring assisted feeding include:

- Anorexic animals (of more than 3 days)
- More than 10% body weight loss
- Physical limitations, e.g. fractured jaw, oral ulceration, facial trauma, etc.
- Following oral surgery – too painful and give tissue time to heal
- Generalised loss of muscle mass
- Generalised lethargy of more than 3 days in severely ill animals
- Megaoesophagus
- Conditions associated with inadequate food intake lasting longer than 3 days

METHODS OF FEEDING

Assess the patient as to what type of feeding is required. Often spending time with an animal gently encouraging it to eat will be enough for the animal to gradually start eating again. There are different ways in which this can be done.

1. ASSISTED AND SYRINGE FEEDING

- Encourage, talk to and stroke the animal
- Warm moist and liquid food to increase the smell and palatability
- Tempt the animal by placing small amounts on its lips, nose, paws, or your fingers
- Clean their face, especially nose and mouth area to enable the animal to smell and breathe whilst eating
- Offer small amounts and one type of food at a time (especially cats)
- Use highly palatable food appropriate for each species, e.g. try oily fish for cats, adding gravy for dogs and soft, sweet fruit and vegetables for rabbits and guinea-pigs
- Fill a small syringe up with liquid food, push the tip through the side of the mouth in between the molars and empty syringe slowly

2. CHEMICALLY ENHANCED ORAL FEEDING

- Diazepam (Valium) may be used in cats as an appetite stimulant. 0.5–1 mg/kg given intravenously as directed by the VS
- This has an immediate effect so make sure the food is already prepared and ready to give as soon as the drug has been administered

3. TUBE FEEDING

Critically ill animals or animals physically unable to eat may require tube feeding. Calculated amounts of food and water are administered via a feeding tube, this ensures that the animal receives adequate nutrition. See Figures 4.1, 4.2 and 4.3. Table 4.1 compares different types of tube feeding.

4. INTRAVENOUS FEEDING (PARENTERAL NUTRITION)

Nutrition may be provided by the intravenous route. Used for patients with gastrointestinal failure (i.e. inflammatory bowel disease, pancreatitis and peritonitis). Special liquids suitable for intravenous administration are used. There is a high risk of infection using this method and so solutions must be mixed aseptically and 24 hour nursing provided.

THE WARD

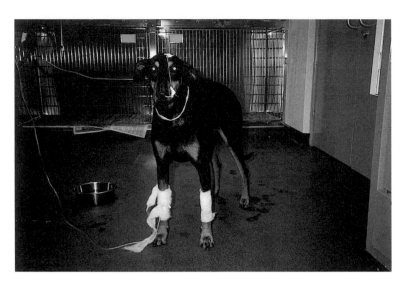

Fig. 4.1 Naso-oesophageal tube in a Doberman dog.

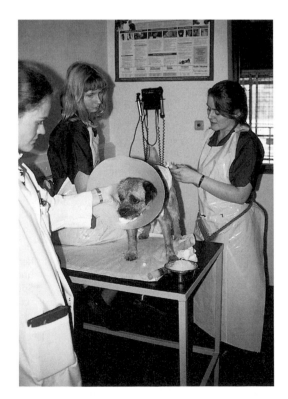

Fig. 4.2   Gastrostomy tube feeding.

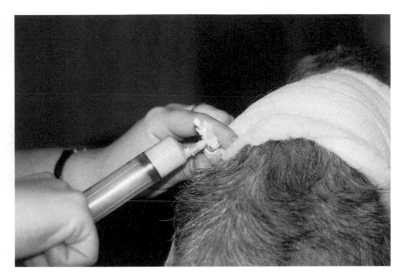

Fig. 4.3 Gastrostomy tube feeding.

Table 4.1 Comparison of types of tube feeding.

Tube	Advantages	Disadvantages
Orogastric (stomach tube)	Useful in neonates and exotics	Not well tolerated by adults Short-term use only
Naso-oesophageal tube The tube is placed via a nostril into the oesophagus (size 3.5–8 French Gauge)	Easy to place Appropriate for up to a week Animal is still able to eat and drink with tube in place	Small gauge tube so only certain liquid feeds can be used
Pharyngostomy tube The tube is placed in the lateral aspect of the pharynx (size 8–18 Fr)	Useful for short- to mid-term use Easy to administer any liquidised food into the oesophagus	Requires general anaesthesia Can be easily dislodged Stoma site can become infected
Gastrostomy tube Placed either endoscopically or via gastrotomy (size 14–20 Fr)	Easy to feed Any liquidised food may be fed Can be left in for months at a time	Requires general anaesthesia Specialised equipment required (endoscope)

CALCULATE THE ENERGY REQUIREMENT

Many hospitalised animals become malnourished because they are not receiving adequate calories as well as a complete nutritional diet.

THE WARD

1. CALCULATE THE BASAL ENERGY REQUIREMENT (BER)

Small dogs and cats (<5 kg)

$$BER = 60 \times (\text{body weight in kg}) \, \text{kcal/day}$$

Dogs over 5 kg

$$BER = 30 \times (\text{body weight in kg}) + 70 \, \text{kcal/day}$$

2. THEN MULTIPLY BY 'DISEASE FACTOR'

Disease factors:

Cage rest: 1.2
Post surgery/trauma: 1.3
Multiple surgery/trauma: 1.5
Sepsis/neoplasia: 1.7
Burns: 2.0
Growth: 2.0

$$BER \times \text{disease factor} = \text{total requirement (kcal/day)}$$

Example
The calorie requirement per day for a 23 kg dog, being hospitalised following a fracture repair of the femur using internal fixation is:

$$30 \times 23 = 690$$

$$690 + 70 = 760$$

$$760 \times 1.3 = 988 \, \text{kcal/day}$$

The hospitalisation factor is taken into consideration in each of the disease processes.

WHAT TO FEED

Depending on whether the food is to be tube fed or not determines the type of food to be used. The more energy dense the diet is the less it is necessary to feed. The following diets (Table 4.2) are often used in assisted and tube feeding.

HOW MUCH TO FEED

Once the type of food to feed has been chosen and the energy requirements of the animal have been calculated it is necessary to calculate how much food the animal requires over the day.

Divide the daily energy requirement by the energy density of the food, which should be stated on the package or tin, to find out the total volume in millilitres per day. If feeding tinned food, it is still possible to work out the required volume by knowing how many kcal/g the food contains.

Daily energy requirement (kcal/day) ÷ energy density (kcal/ml) of the food = amount in ml to feed

Table 4.2 Comparisons of different types of food.

Type	Energy density	Characteristics
Whiskas Feline & Pedigree Canine Liquid Concentrate™ (Waltham)	Whiskas™ 1.2 kcal/ml Pedigree™ 1.5 kcal/ml	Powder form mixed with water to correct dilution Suitable for most sizes of naso-oesophageal tubes Palatable for assisted feeding
Hill's Pet Nutrition a/d™	1.3 kcal/ml	Semi-liquid food For tubes > 8 French Gauge Palatable for assisted feeding
Eukanuba Nutritional Recovery™	2.1 kcal/ml	Semi-liquid food For tubes > 8 French Gauge Palatable for assisted feeding
Reanimyl™	0.9 kcal/ml	Liquid food suitable for all tube feeding especially naso-oesophageal tubes Not very palatable for assisted feeding
Ensure™	1.5 kcal/ml	Human product available in different flavours (vanilla is probably most appropriate) Suitable for naso-oesophageal tubes Nutritional quality not totally appropriate for animals so long-term use not recommended

THE WARD

Example

An animal requires 1050 kcal per day and the energy density of the chosen food is 1.2 kcal/ml.

$$1050 \, kcal \div 1.2 \, kcal/ml = 875 \, ml \text{ per day}$$

This amount may then be divided up into smaller meals to be fed throughout the day.

TUBE FEEDING

CONTINUOUS FEEDING

- Via drip bag or syringe pump at 1 ml/kg/hour
- Gradually increase until daily volume can be fed over 12–18 hrs

REPEATED BOLUS

- Give a calculated quantity divided throughout the day.
- Give up to 30–45 ml/kg per feed. The stomach capacity is 50–90 ml/kg (but is reduced following periods of inappetance).

HOW TO FEED USING A NASO-OESOPHAGEAL TUBE

(1) Place a few drops of local anaesthetic around the tube into the nostril about 5 minutes before the feed. This prevents the animal being irritated by any movement of the tube as it is fed.

(2) Warm the food to body temperature.

(3) If it is not certain whether the tube is in place flush first with 1–2 ml of sterile saline or radiograph patient.

(4) Flush the tube with 5–10 ml of water (warm).

(5) Slowly administer the required amount of food. Use 20 ml syringes as less force is required to syringe the food.

(6) Observe the animal, ensuring it is showing no signs of discomfort.

(7) After administering the food flush the tube again with water to clear the tube of food.

(8) Increase the amount gradually starting with one-third daily allowance over the first day.

(9) For the 24 hours, dilute the food by 50% to reduce the chance of diarrhoea.

HOW TO FEED USING A GASTROSTOMY TUBE

(1) Do not use for first 24 hours, allowing time for a primary seal to form between the stomach and body wall.

(2) Start with small amounts of water (5 ml/kg) to flush the tube.

(3) At first, feed only a third of the daily requirements divided into several small meals. Increase to normal amount over 3 days.

(4) Ensure the food is warmed to body temperature and administer slowly, observing the animal for any signs of discomfort.

(5) Always flush the tube after feeding.

(6) Check placement of tube and clean wound if necessary.

(7) Replace the bandage over the feeding tube.

CARE OF FEEDING TUBES

- Radiograph to ensure correct positioning of distal end of tube (most naso-oesophageal tubes have a radio-opaque line).
- Test the tube each feed by syringing 1–2 ml of sterile saline (if it goes into the trachea, the saline will be absorbed quickly). If the animal coughs, check the position as shown above.
- Always flush tubes after feeding to prevent clogging of tube with food.
- Replace spigot after use.
- Unclog blocked tubes by flushing with water or fizzy drink – the bubbles will help break down the blockage.
- Check tube entry site daily and cover with dressing and bandage if necessary (gastrostomy tubes and pharyngostomy).
- Prevent patient interference with Elizabethan collar or bandage.
- Check patient for evidence of vomiting, regurgitation or bloating.

THE WARD

• Check for diarrhoea.
• Check body weight daily.
• In the event of aspiration of food, stop feeding, report to the VS and remove the tube.

FLUID INTAKE

If the animal is drinking unaided, it is easy to calculate the total quantity of fluids that the animal is consuming by placing a measured amount in a nonspill bowl and then measuring what is left at a later time. All details must be recorded on a chart such as the one shown in Table 4.3.

If the animal's intake does not match daily requirements, additional methods of providing rehydration will be required. (Do not forget to consider quantity of water in any food given). Repeated forced application of oral fluids is not recommended, as it is stressful for the animal.

ORAL REHYDRATION PRODUCTS

• Pedigree Electrolyte Instant Fluid™
• Lectade™

Oral rehydration therapy is used to treat mild dehydration and electrolyte losses. These sachets contain powders, which are combined with water and given orally as a liquid solution.

Table 4.3   Example of a water intake chart.

Day	Time	Quantity given	Time checked	Quantity left	Amount consumed	Comments
1/2/01	9 AM	500 ml	2 PM	475 ml	25 ml	
1/2/01	2 PM	500 ml	10 PM	480 ml	20 ml	
1/2/01	10 PM	500 ml	8 AM	450 ml	50 ml	
2/2/01	8 AM	500 ml				

CHAPTER 5

CLEANING AND GROOMING THE PATIENT

Grooming and cleaning the patient is important to promote well-being. It also gets the animal used to being handled in the veterinary practice, thereby reducing the patient's fear and anxiety and helps to build up trust between nurse and patient.

Medically, it is important for hygiene reasons. Removal of dirt, crusts and loose hair contributes towards the health of the animals and will make it less likely that abnormalities are overlooked.

For most hospitalised patients, grooming and cleaning should be part of the every day ward procedure. (Those with heart disorders; respiratory distress and zoonotic diseases should *only* be groomed with the veterinary surgeon's consent.) It is better to spend a few minutes grooming regularly than many hours sporadically.

Whilst not a professional groomer, the VN should be aware of some of the different coat types in dog and cat breeds and the grooming equipment most suited to their hair type.

The coat is made up of two main types of hair:

• Guard hairs – rigid primary hairs
• Lanugo hairs – soft, thinner hairs

The type of coat an animal has is governed by the combination of these hairs (see Tables 5.1 and 5.2).

Most cats do not require bathing and on the whole, only show cats get bathed regularly. Unless the cat likes water, it's usually an extremely stressful time for both the cat and the owner, and drying them with a hair dryer is nearly impossible.

Table 5.1   General care for different coat types in dogs.

Type of coat	Example of breeds	Special tools/ equipment	Technique
Long coat	Newfoundland, GSD, Old English Sheep Dog, Collie, Siberian Husky, Samoyed, Corgi	Rake. Bristle/wire brush. Fine Resco comb	Rake dead hair, comb and brush forward over top and sides, backward over flanks. Fine-comb chin, tail and ears
Silky coat	Spaniel, Afghan, Maltese, Yorkshire Terrier, Setter, Lhasa Apso, Peke	Wire brush. Medium and fine steel combs. Bristle brushes	Frequent bathing to prevent mats. Spaniels need stripping every 3 months
Nonshedding curly/woolly	Poodle, Bedlington Terrier, Kerry Blue	Oster clippers no. 7, 10 and 15 blades. Natural bristle brush. Steel combs	Clip every 4–8 weeks. Comb and brush to prevent mats
Smooth coat	Doberman, Retriever, Boxer, Dachshund, Dalmatian, Beagle	Hound glove. Rubber brush	Rub coat for sleekness and to remove dead hairs
Wiry coat	Fox Terrier, Welsh Terrier, Airedale, Lakeland Terrier, Schnauzer, Sealyham	Oster clippers no. 7, 10 and 15. Duplex stripping knife, slicker brush, hound glove	Hand strip and brush with slicker and hound glove to remove dead hair
Corded coat	Komondor, Puli	Shampoo – diluted 10:1 in a water spray. Hair dryer	Never clip or comb. Bath if dirty. Squeeze dry – do not brush or rub coat when wet

Table 5.2   General care for different coat types in cats.

Type of coat	Example of breeds	Special tools/ equipment	Technique
Short-haired single coat	Siamese, Burmese, Havana Brown, Rex, Korat, Domestic Short Hair	Fine metal comb, natural boar bristle brush	Shampoo and water if necessary. Brush and comb against coat to remove dead hair
Short-haired double coat	Abyssinian, Manx, Russian Blue, American Shorthaired	As above	Similar to above. Avoid excessive grooming – it destroys the coat
Long-haired	Persians, Himalayans	Several sizes of metal combs. Boar bristle brush	Shampoo and water and dry quickly. Daily brush and comb

GROOMING EQUIPMENT

Use combs with care. The metal teeth can scratch and bruise the skin very badly. Forced combing or pulling at tangled mats pulls out both live and dead hairs and causes discomfort, pain, irritation and secondary bacterial infection of the skin. It also ruins the coat.

A *slicker* or *carder* may be used to loosen the coat and remove the dead hair. They are useful on smaller hair mats and for general grooming purposes. They may cause injury to areas of the body with sparse hair covering, so use with care.

Natural *bristle brushes* are considered preferable to nylon bristles because they cause less static electricity, which can cause hair breakage. These brushes are useful on very short hair only because they do not get down to the hair near the skin, so it remains matted whilst the top layer looks fine.

Hound gloves are used on short-haired breeds to remove the dead undercoat and give the coat a shine.

Stripping combs have a razor blade or serrated metal blade encased in teeth. These are used to help pull out dead hair. The hair is grasped between the thumb and the comb and removed with a twisting motion.

Hand stripping or plucking is a technique used by some owners and groomers to remove hairs.

PREPARATION FOR BATHING

- Before dogs are bathed, their coats should be brushed out and their claws clipped
- Hair from inbetween the pads can be trimmed using clippers if possible (safer than scissors)
- Severe mats and tangles should be cut out before they are wet because they become much more difficult to remove after they have become wet
- The anal sacs should be palpated and expressed if necessary
- The ears should be examined
- Pledgets of cotton wool may be placed into each ear before bathing to prevent soap and water entering and causing irritation
- Do not apply any ointments or oils to the eyes (this used to be popular; however, it is more difficult to rinse an irritant from the eye)

Select shampoo agent suitable for each particular case. (See Table 5.3.)

THE WARD

Table 5.3   Shampoos and their uses.

Product name	Active principle(s)	Uses
Deocare™ Shampoo	Shampoo	Cleansing and deodorising
Derasect Insecticidal and Conditioning Shampoo™	Carbaryl	Routine use to restore natural lustre and to control fleas
Epi-soothe™	Colloidal oatmeal	Pruritis
Etiderm™	Ethyl lactate, benzyl alcohol	Bacterial skin infection
Hexocil™	Hexetidine 0.5%	Shampoo and conditioning
Malaseb™	Chlorhexidine and miconazole	Treatment of fungal or yeast infections
Oxydex™	Benzoyl peroxide	Canine dermatitis, pyoderma, sebhorrhoeic dermatitis
Paxcutol™	Benzolyl peroxide 2.5%	Bacterial skin infection and/or seborrhoea
Sebocalm™	Olefin sulphonate, lauramide DEA, glycerine	Normal and dry skin
Sebolytic™	Coal tar, sulphur, salicylic acid	Greasy seborrhoea
Seleen™	Selenium sulphide 1%	Seborrhoeic dermatitis
Tarlite™	3% jupicol tar, 2% sulphur, 2% salicylic acid	Canine seborrhoea, dry skin

BATHING PROCEDURE

(1) Thoroughly wet skin surface with warm water.

(2) Use a sponge to wet skin around face and difficult to reach areas.

(3) Apply shampoo at several points over body.

(4) Gently massage into coat and skin all over the dog until sufficient shampoo is used to produce a good lather (use manufacturer's recommendations).

(5) Take care around the face area to avoid eyes, nose, mouth and ears.

(6) Leave shampoo on for contact time if necessary.

(7) Thoroughly rinse all of the shampoo from the skin using large amounts of warm water.

(8) Squeeze the coat to remove excess water and allow the dog to shake itself.

(9) Thoroughly dry with hand towels.

(10) Gently comb the hair, taking care not to pull mats.

(11) Dry dog using a blow dryer. Take care never to hold the dryer in one place for too long and do not hold too close to the skin.

CLIPPING CLAWS

(1) Assistant to restrain patient
(2) Take hold of the foot using the same hand; push each toe to expose the nail fully
(3) If the quick is visible, place the clippers distally to the quick and cut the nail at an angle with a rapid action
(4) If the quick is not visible (black claws), apply slight pressure with the clippers at an estimated position
(5) If the animal reacts badly, reposition the clippers further distally and try again, clipping as before
(6) Clip each nail in turn, not forgetting to check for dewclaws, these are often very overgrown and can easily be hidden in long-haired coats.
(7) If bleeding occurs, press a piece of cotton wool against the end of the nail and if bleeding persists apply a silver nitrate pencil or friar's balsam styptic
(8) Always ensure that the patient is restrained properly and talked to throughout the procedure

It is advisable to offer treats during and after the process to make future attempts easier.

SQUEEZING ANAL GLANDS

(1) Assistant is required to restrain the dog, as it may be uncomfortable
(2) Put on examination gloves
(3) Apply generous amount of lubricant (liquid paraffin, KY™ gel) to index finger
(4) Insert lubricated finger into rectum and locate full sacs. They are located at 4 o'clock and 8 o'clock and vary in size (usually about pea size when full)
(5) Gently squeeze contents of the sac dorsomedially between the finger and thumb.
(6) Use cotton wool to wipe sac contents away from around the anus
(7) Holding the cotton wool in the same hand as the one used to express, remove the glove by inverting it and tying it in a knot to reduce the smell left in the room
(8) Wipe some animal deodorising spray (e.g. Petfresh™) around the area to leave fresher smell

CLIPPING BEAKS

Beak overgrowth is common in small psittacines such as cock-atiels and budgerigars. It is usually due to malocclusion, which prevents the beaks wearing down in the normal way. These birds will require their beaks to be trimmed regularly. This may be done using bone forceps, file or fine nail clippers.

Care must be taken not to cut the sensitive structures under the keratin, as this may cause infection or growth abnormality.

After trimming the beak should be smoothed with sandpaper or a file.

CLIPPING FLIGHT FEATHERS

Some owners of psittacines want to stop their bird from flying, however, it is important to advise them that clipping the flight feathers does not necessarily stop them flying completely and many birds may be able to fly short distances even when the flight feathers have been cut properly. Clipping one wing only will help to reduce their aerodynamic lift and prevent sustained flight.

Each primary feather should be cut just below the level of the covert feathers so that the trimmed end is not visible. The last three distal primary feathers should be left uncut (Fig. 5.1).

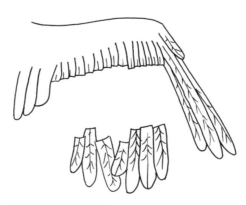

THE LAST 3 FEATHERS
SHOULD BE LEFT UNCUT
SO THAT THE WING
LOOKS MORE
NATURAL WHEN
FOLDED UP IN ITS
RESTING POSITION

Fig. 5.1   Clipping flight feathers

Feathers that are in their growing phase should not be cut because they will bleed profusely.

New feathers will eventually grow and replace the cut feathers. The rate of growth is irregular, but generally, the wings may be clipped once a year.

THE WARD

CHAPTER 6

DRESSINGS AND BANDAGES

A VN should be proficient in all bandaging techniques ensuring that appropriate dressings are used. New products are always being developed as well as new techniques for wound management.

THE CONTACT LAYER (PRIMARY WOUND DRESSING)

There are many ways to classify wound-dressing materials. For example, the following terms may be used:

- Dry dressings
- Moist dressings
- Wet dressings
- Impregnated gauze
- Adherent or nonadherent dressings

It is important that the VN knows what is available and what is most appropriate for a particular wound at each stage of its healing process.

DRY DRESSINGS (NONADHERENT)

Generally, dry dressings such as Melolin™, may be used on surgical wounds where the edges of the wound are held together. For most other types of wound, they have been shown to be detrimental to wound healing. They tend to adhere to the wound surface, causing pain and disruption of the healing processes upon removal.

Dry to dry

This method of dry to dry dressings has gone out of fashion. Their main application is for dirty, necrotic wounds that have lots of loose tissue and foreign matter to remove. Sterile surgical gauze is applied dry to the wound surface. When it is removed (each day), a layer of tissue is removed along with the necrotic material and debris.

The main reason for their discontinued use is that removal can be extremely uncomfortable, if not painful, for the patient and it is not just the necrotic tissue and debris that is removed. A certain amount of the healthy, healing cells are disrupted and removed. This type of dressing should never be used in wounds with good granulation and epithelialisation.

Wet to dry

Wet to dry work in a very similar way to dry to dry dressings. The gauze swab is first soaked in sterile saline before being applied to the wound. This reduces the viscosity of wound exudate so that it may be absorbed more easily. The fluid then evaporates and the dressing becomes dry by the time it is removed thus pulling away everything else with it.

These dressings have added disadvantages over dry to dry because the moist environment is conducive to bacterial growth. In addition, the tissues surrounding the wound may become macerated if the dressing is too wet. The use of cold wetting solutions can cause discomfort to the animal.

Impregnated gauze dressings

These are slightly less adherent than dry dressings but they do very little to actively promote wound healing. Examples include Jelonet™ and Grassolind™.

Poultice

A poultice is a paste or impregnated dressing that is applied to an area to draw out infection. Poultices are used more widely in large animal medicine than for small animals. Animalintex™ is the most commonly used commercial poultice.

MOIST DRESSINGS (NONADHERENT)

Moist wound dressings (hydrogels such as Intrasite™ and Biodres™ and hydrophilics such as Allevyn™) are interactive dressing materials that are extremely useful in maintaining a moist wound environment. Their use has been shown to accelerate wound healing by providing an optimum wound temperature, encourage the migration of cells from the edges of the wound and encouraging cell mitosis. They remove excess exudate and toxic components whilst giving protection from

THE WARD

secondary infection. They are easy to remove and do not cause trauma or pain at dressing change.

Note: there is no single dressing material that can provide the optimum environment for all wounds or for the total healing stages of one wound, therefore it is important to select the most appropriate dressing for each wound at each particular stage of the healing process. This is why it is important for the VN to research available products and keep up to date with new materials.

APPLICATION OF BANDAGES

A bandage should consist of three layers; each layer having its own distinct characteristics and functions:

PRIMARY DRESSING (OR CONTACT LAYER)

- Sterile
- Must remain in close contact with the wound
- Allow drainage of exudate
- Prevent contamination from environment

Examples: Melolin™, Intrasite Gel™, Allevyn™, Rondo-pad™.

SECONDARY (OR INTERMEDIATE PADDING LAYER)

- Absorb fluids
- Provide padding
- Provide comfort and immobilisation

Examples: Cotton wool, Soffban™, Ortho-band™.

TERTIARY (OUTER LAYER)

- Secures other dressings/bandages in place
- Provides additional support and protection
- Protects other dressings/bandages from getting dirty

Examples:
    Cohesive bandages: Co-Form™, Co-Flex™, Powerflex™.
    Adhesive bandages: Bandesive™, E-Band™, Elastoplast™, Treatplast™.

RULES OF BANDAGING

(1) Collect all necessary equipment first. See Fig. 6.1
(2) Ensure the animal is adequately restrained
(3) *Always* wash hands prior to handling and wear sterile gloves if necessary
(4) Apply layers evenly, prevent areas of excess pressure (hocks, elbows)
(5) Do not unroll too much bandage at a time
(6) A bandage on a swollen limb will become loose once swelling has subsided
(7) Avoid sticking too much adhesive to fur (remove with alcohol)
(8) For fractures: include proximal and distal joints to adequately immobilise the fracture
(9) Check that the bandage is not too tight: it should be possible to insert two fingers between the bandage and the animal
(10) Change dressings as often as necessary, and check frequently

In the presence of an infected wound, the VN should wear gloves and a protective apron to maintain personal hygiene and health.

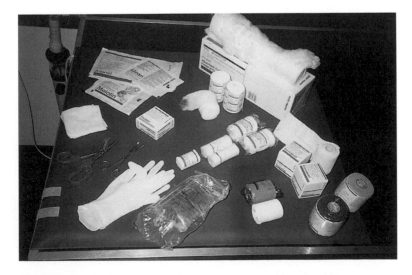

Fig. 6.1 Bandaging equipment.

THE WARD

PREVENTION OF SELF-TRAUMA

Animals may try to remove a dressing or bandage if it is uncomfortable or painful. Check if this is the problem before trying methods of prevention.

Methods

- Elizabethan (Buster™) collars, see Fig. 6.2
- Neck braces (Bite Not™), see Fig. 6.3
- Bandages (or old T-shirts, socks, etc.)
- Topical applications (Bitter apple or Tabasco sauce)
- Sedation

PRESSURE BANDAGES

- Used to control haemorrhage and prevent excess swelling and oedema
- *Remove* after 12–24 hours, as it will reduce drainage to the tissues
- Change if animal appears uncomfortable

Avoid excess padding on convex surfaces, as this increases the pressure in this area.

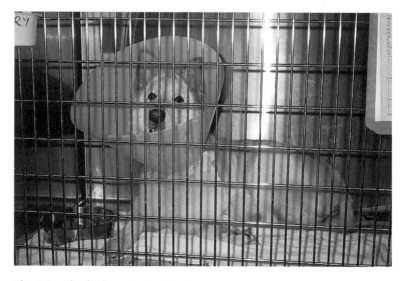

Fig. 6.2   Elizabethan (Buster™) collar.

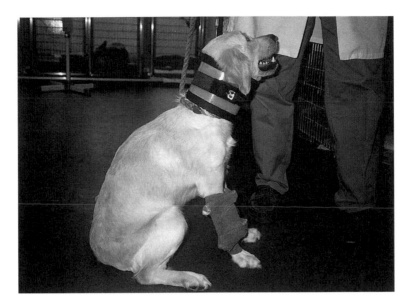

Fig. 6.3 Neck braces (Bite Not™).

Make sure that pressure bandages are marked so everyone is aware of them and knows when they should be removed.

AFTER-CARE OF BANDAGES AND CLIENT INFORMATION

It must be stressed to owners (and hospital lay staff) that the success of treatment depends on good care of the animal's dressing and bandage. The VN or client must inform the VS if any of the following occurs:

- Bandage begins to smell
- Bandage slips from original position
- Areas of soreness develop around the bandage
- Discharge seeps through the bandage
- Persistent patient interference

It is important to keep the bandage both clean and dry. When the animal is being taken outside, the lower part of the bandage should be covered with a plastic bag or empty drip bag and secured with a piece of tape or loose elastic band. The bag *must* be removed as soon as the pet is back inside or the foot will sweat.

THE WARD

BANDAGING TECHNIQUES

USEFUL TIPS FOR BANDAGE APPLICATION

- 'Stirrups' will help prevent limb bandages slipping down the limb and are useful for most limb bandages (the tapes should not be applied over wounds or areas with skin lesions)
- Avoid sticking adhesive bandages to the fur if possible, they pull the hairs causing discomfort, which frequently results in the patient chewing or interfering with the bandage
- Always unroll bandage as shown in Fig. 6.4, this prevents the operator 'running out' of bandage
- When bandaging a limb, start distally and work proximately, rather than working down the limb

Forelimb/hindlimb bandage
Used to hold wound dressings in position; postoperatively for support and to help control inflammation, and as a first aid support measure for fracture management. See Fig. 6.4.

- Check length of claws, clip if necessary
- Cover any wounds with an appropriate dressing
- Cotton wool between toes and pads, do not forget dew claw
- Position joints in natural angles, do not over-extend limb
- Apply synthetic padding bandage layer or cotton wool around the limb
- Apply splint if required
- Apply conforming bandage to the distal limb first before winding evenly up the limb overlapping the previous layer by half the bandage width

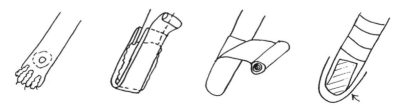

Fig. 6.4   Type of bandage used for fore or hindlimb.

- Separate distal ends of the tape strips and turn over and extend up along the proximal bandage to adhere to the conforming layer
- Place protective layer of cohesive bandage or adhesive bandage over the top

Ear and head bandage
Used to control haemorrhage from pinnae, for aural resection and aural haematoma.

- Apply dressing to wound
- Place pad of cotton wool on top of head
- Fold ear back onto pad and cover with further padding
- Apply conforming bandage over the top passing either side of the free ear in a figure-of-eight pattern, see Fig. 6.5
- Cover with cohesive outer layer
- Make sure that the bandage layers are not applied too tightly, it should be possible to slip two fingers underneath the bandage easily and the patient should be able to breath easily and open its mouth
- Draw over the top with felt-tipped pen the position of the covered ear to prevent cutting through the pinna when removing

Abdominal bandage
Used following abdominal surgery or trauma, to hold wound

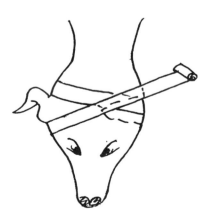

Fig. 6.5 Ear and head bandage.

drain in place or to hold gastrostomy tube in place. (See Fig. 6.6.)

- Cover wound or incision with dressing
- Use minimal padding – enough for comfort; too much will cause the bandage to slip
- Use wide conforming bandage followed by a cohesive (Elastoplast is too restrictive)
- You may include the forelegs or hindlegs to prevent slipping or 'bunching' up.

Thoracic bandage

Used following surgery or trauma, and to retain chest drain.

- Cover wound or incision with dressing
- Use minimal padding
- Use wide conforming bandage
- Cover with cohesive bandage *not* elastic adhesive
- Include forelegs in figure-of-eight fashion to anchor bandage, see Fig. 6.7

Tail bandage

Used following tip amputation to prevent further trauma.

- May use similar method to limb bandage – but with less padding
- Stent dressing – swab is sutured to end of tail

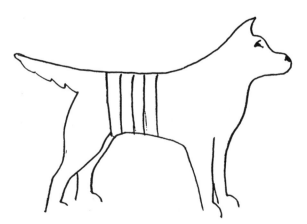

Fig. 6.6 Abdominal bandage.

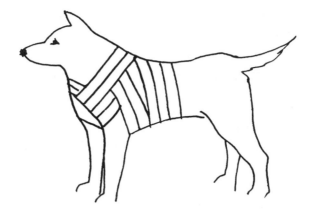

Fig. 6.7 Thoracic bandage.

- Syringe case is adapted to fit over the end and then secured to the tail

Robert Jones bandage

Used as a first aid support, to immobilise a fractured limb and to give additional support following joint surgery.

- Apply traction tapes to dorsal and ventral surfaces of lower limb
- Unroll cotton wool from roll and wrap firmly around the limb
- Cover first padding layer with conforming bandage
- Repeat layers of cotton wool at least two more times
- Incorporate traction tapes into layers to prevent slipping
- Cover bandage with Elastoplast™ or cohesive outer layer
- Leave distal end of middle two toes free in order to check circulation

Ehmer sling

Used to prevent dislocation of hip joint. See Fig. 6.8.

- Place animal in lateral recumbency with affected leg uppermost
- Apply padding to metatarsus and stifle
- Flex the leg and rotate the foot inwards
- Apply conforming bandage to the metatarsus bringing it medial to the stifle

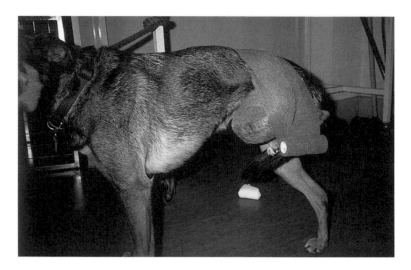

Fig. 6.8   Ehmer sling.

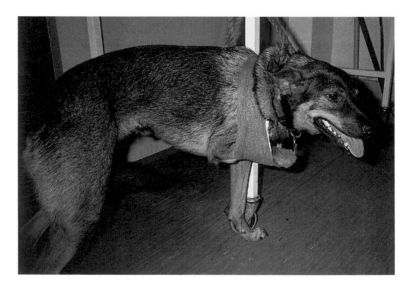

Fig. 6.9   Velpeau sling.

- Continue over thigh, behind the hock and back to the meta-tarsus in a figure-of-eight pattern
- The whole bandage may then be strapped to the body using cohesive tape

Velpeau sling
Used to support and immobilise the shoulder joint. See Fig. 6.9.

- Apply layer of padding material to the foreleg
- Hold the paw in flexion and apply the bandage from the paw, over the back of the animal behind the other foreleg and back to the flexed paw
- Continue in this fashion to stabilise the limb
- Cover with adhesive or cohesive bandage

THE WARD

CHAPTER 7

PHYSIOTHERAPY

Massage provides the easiest method of physiotherapy and no specialised equipment is required. The primary objectives of massage are:

- Speed up healing of injured tissues
- Help restore normal function
- Help prevent disability
- Decrease hospitalisation time

This may be achieved by:

- Increasing blood flow through the massaged tissues
- Enhancing lymph flow
- Decreasing fibrosis
- Reducing oedema
- Reducing muscle spasm
- Stretching contractions

Other methods of physiotherapy include:

- Hydrotherapy, see Fig. 7.1
- Supported movement, see Figs 7.2, 7.3 and 7.4
- Heat and cold therapy

Massage may be used for:

- Tight contracted tendons, ligaments and muscles
- Chronic inflammatory conditions
- Peripheral nerve injuries
- Scar tissue
- Acute and chronic oedema

Massage should not be performed in the presence of:

- Acute inflammation
- Fractures or sprains
- Haemorrhage

- Metastatic disease
- Infections

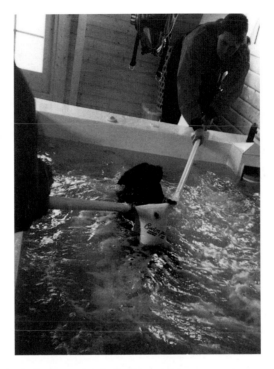

Fig. 7.1   Physiotherapy using hydrotherapy.

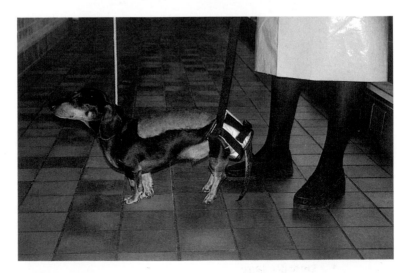

Fig. 7.2   Assisting a paraplegic dog by using a harness.

THE WARD

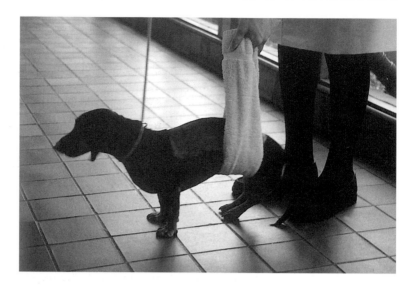

Fig. 7.3   Assisting a paraplegic dog by using a towel as a sling.

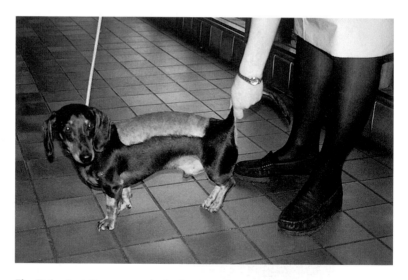

Fig. 7.4   Assisting a paraplegic dog to walk.

PHYSIOTHERAPY TECHNIQUES

There are five basic techniques:

- Effleurage
- Petrissage
- Friction

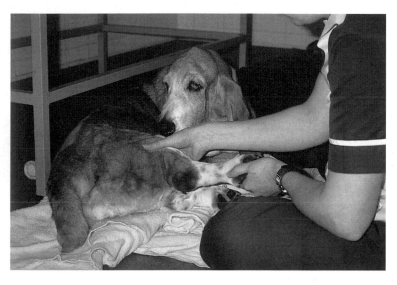

Fig. 7.5 Massaging a dog.

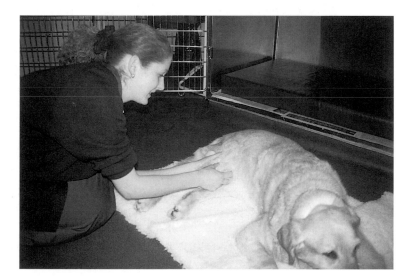

Fig.7.6 Massaging a dog.

- Passive joint movement
- Active movement

See Figs 7.5 and 7.6.

Lubricants (e.g. olive oil, soft white paraffin or baby powder) may be used to soften the skin and reduce friction. These agents should not be applied to wounds. Massage should be 10–30 minutes long each day. Whichever type of massage is most appropriate, always start each session with effleurage as a warm up to the main session.

EFFLEURAGE

This is a gentle massage technique, which precedes the other three types. Effleurage accustoms the animal to touch and warms up the underlying tissues. The hands work using a light or heavy stroke with uniform pressure. The patient is massaged from the periphery of the limb or affected area to the centre. A light stroke at a rate of 15 strokes per minute applied for a sedative effect. A heavy stroke at a rate of five strokes per minute is applied to enhance draining of lymph channels. This part of the session should last approximately 10 minutes to prepare the patient for more extensive massage using one or more of the following techniques depending on the animal's condition.

PETRISSAGE (KNEADING OR COMPRESSION)

Used primarily on muscles to enhance circulation and stretch muscles, tendons, adhesions and contractions. The muscle is compressed from side to side as the hands move up the muscle – always in the direction of venous return. The pressure should be gentle and never forceful enough to cause pain.

FRICTION

Used to aid the absorption of local effusions and loosen superficial scar tissue and adhesions. Skin is moved over the underlying tissue in small, circular, rhythmic motions while pressure is applied across the tendon or adhesion to encourage collagen formation. Should only last 3–7 minutes.

PASSIVE MOVEMENT

Used to retain and/or regain joint mobility. The affected joint is held above and below and put through its normal range of motion. This should be done no more than ten times on each joint three to five times a day. Never perform passive movement on a joint that has not been warmed up first and always prepare the area using effleurage first to warm up the joint and prevent pain on manipulation.

ACTIVE MOVEMENT

Active movement involves voluntary activity by the patient. It can be started with gentle pulling on the toes and encouraging the patient to pull them away. For paraplegics, loop a towel or harness under the abdomen and support, whilst encouraging the patient to weight bear on the hind limbs. The patient may be walked around to maintain muscle tone in the front limbs. The total time spent on harness walking will depend on the individual case, but generally 10 minutes three times daily is adequate.

OTHER TECHNIQUES

COUPAGE

This is used to clear any secretions from the airway (hypostatic congestion) by gentle percussion of the thorax using cupped hands. Always work from the caudal end of the chest to the cranial end, this will encourage coughing and the removal of secretions. Always percuss both sides of the thorax. Coupage should be performed *gently* and not cause lung damage. See Fig. 7.7.

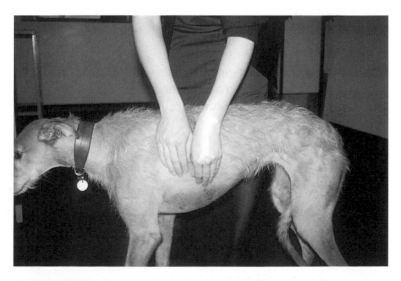

Fig. 7.7 Performing coupage.

HYDROTHERAPY

The physical properties of water buoyancy and hydrostatic pressure provide support. The patient should be immersed into a bath or whirlpool that is just too deep for the animal to stand and be supported by the handler while swimming, see Fig. 7.1. Water movement (by means of a shower head attachment can be added to create a massage effect). The water temperature should be 38.8°–40.5°C (102°–105°F). Povidone-iodine or similar can be added to the water to help prevent any skin infections from decubital ulcers or urinary scalds. Animals must never be left alone in the water. Some animals will need reassurance and encouragement to ease fear. Always dry the patient thoroughly following bathing.

COLD THERAPY

Application of cold to an area causes vasoconstriction, which helps to reduce inflammation and provide mild analgesia.
Indicated to:

- Reduce/prevent oedema
- Treat burns
- Decrease swelling
- Reduce muscle spasms

Contra-indicated in:

- Open wounds
- Fractures

This therapy is usually used as *a first aid measure immediately following a traumatic injury*. Various cold packs may be used including:

- Commercial cold packs
- Packets of frozen vegetables
- A latex glove filled with very cold water
- Pieces of ice placed into leak-proof plastic bags

All types of ice packs should be wrapped inside a towel to protect the animal's skin and should be applied for 5–20 minutes.

HEAT THERAPY

Heat therapy is useful for its analgesic properties. Heat helps to reduce muscle stiffness, muscle spasms and promotes wound healing. Its application is also useful:

- Postoperatively
- Relieving stiff joints
- Relieving muscle stiffness
- Following trauma

It should not be used for patients with decreased sensation, e.g. neurological patients and in acute inflammatory conditions.

Methods of applying heat include:

- Commercial heat packs
- Hot water bottle wrapped in a towel
- Heat pads
- Drip bags heated in the microwave
- Bags of corn heated in the microwave

CONTRAST BATHING

This technique is usually used after the time has elapsed where cold therapy will no longer be effective. It is an excellent method of increasing circulatory flow, decreasing swelling, contusions and speeding the elimination of tissue exudate.

Apply ice pack for 3 minutes followed by a heat pack for 3 minutes. Repeat this procedure for 20–30 minutes.

THE WARD

CHAPTER 8

ADMINISTRATION AND DISPENSING OF MEDICATIONS

One of the responsibilities of the VN in the practice is the preparation of medications prescribed by the VS and ensuring that inpatients receive the correct dose at the correct time.

Before administering or dispensing any medications the VN must check the following:

(1) The dose
(2) The dosage interval
(3) The route of administration

Altering one of these components may result in drug concentrations that are too high or too low.

1. THE DOSE

The dose of a drug varies depending on the manufacturer. For this reason, the VN must always state the dose of a drug in units of mass, such as the milligrams or grams rather than the number of products or volume (millilitre, ml).

For example, writing 3 ml of xylazine (Rompun™) is unacceptable because it comes in concentrations of 20 mg/ml and 100 mg/ml. Therefore, 3 ml could contain either 60 mg of the drug or 300 mg. In many cases such an error could be fatal.

The calculation to find out an amount is:

Dose prescribed (mg) ÷ Concentration (mg/ml)

For example, a 20 kg dog needs 20 mg/kg of ampicillin. The ampicillin comes as a concentration of 100 mg/ml

$$20 \times 20 = 400\,mg$$

$$400 \div 100 = 4\,ml$$

2. THE DOSAGE INTERVAL

The time between drug dosages is often expressed using Latin abbreviations and it is essential that the VN is fully aware of them. Commonly used terms:

SID   Once daily (every 24 hrs)
BID   Twice daily (every 12 hrs)
TID   Three times daily (every 8 hrs)
QID   Four times daily (every 6 hrs)
Q4h   Every four hours
o.d.   Every day
e.o.d. Every two days (every other day)
Prn   As needed

The dosage interval may be adjusted to suit either the client or hospital staffing times and still give the required amount over a 24-hour period. However, drug manufacturers recommend certain dosage intervals for each drug and as near as possible these should be adhered to. Some drugs *must* be given at certain intervals to ensure adequate and continuous levels of the drug in the body, for example, phenobarbitone. Changes should only be made under the direction of the VS.

3. ROUTES OF ADMINISTRATION

Unless given by their correct route of administration, the amount of drug that reaches the target tissues in the body can be dramatically reduced or altered. Once again, every drug manufacturer will recommend the suitable route for each drug. The general classification for drug administration is as follows:

- Oral administration (per os): drugs given by mouth
- Parenteral administration: drugs given by injection
- Topical administration: drugs applied to the surface of the body

Table 8.1 shows different routes for administering drugs.

CORRECT PROCEDURE TO REMOVE DRUGS FROM

MULTIDOSE BOTTLES

(1) Check 'best before' date on bottle (discard if out of date)

Table 8.1   Different routes for administering drugs.

Route	Site	Notes
Oral	By mouth	Convenient – may be carried out by owner at home Slower and less complete than by injection Not recommended for vomiting patients Drug may be unstable or destroyed in gastric acid Food present in the gastrointestinal tract may slow absorption
Parenteral -Subcutaneous	Area of loose skin – 'scruff'	Only non-irritant drugs should be used as local irritation may occur. Absorption is much slower as there is a poor blood supply to the area. Depending on the drug, effect will take place 30–45 minutes after injection. Large volumes of fluid may be injected subcutaneously
-Intravenous	Cephalic Lateral saphenous Jugular	Drug is introduced directly into the bloodstream so fastest effect. May be administered in one 'bolus' or slowly as I/V infusion over several seconds, minutes or even hours. Always inject I/V solutions slowly. Drugs that are irritant to tissues are preferably injected I/V
-Intramuscular	Quadriceps Lumbodorsal Trapezius Triceps	The hamstring and gluteals should be avoided due to close proximity of the sciatic nerve. Large amounts of fluid may be painful if injected intramuscularly (max. 5 ml in dogs, 2 ml in cats) Depending on the drug, effect will take place 20–30 minutes after injection
Topical	Skin Ears Eyes Mucous membranes	*Skin* Some drugs may be absorbed through the skin to provide a systemic effect If taken orally, the liver effectively removes it from the system before it can take effect *Mucous membranes* Some drugs are easily absorbed through the mucous membranes (nose, eyes, and mouth) to produce systemic effects

(2) Check the contents of bottle for cloudiness or foreign particles (discard if present)

(3) Clean rubber cap with isopropyl alcohol (except insulin and vaccines)

(4) Insert a 19 g needle into cap to vent the bottle and prevent pressure differentials

(5) Insert syringe needle and invert the vial

(6) Withdraw the prescribed amount of drug

(7) Remove syringe needle from bottle

(8) Replace needle guard and tap the syringe to dislodge any air bubbles

(9) Expel air from syringe

(10) Remove 19 g needle from bottle and discard into sharps box

SINGLE-DOSE AMPOULES

(1) Check 'best before' date on box of ampoules (discard if out of date)

(2) Check the solution for cloudiness or foreign particles (discard if present)

(3) Tap the neck of the ampoule gently to ensure that all of the solution is in the bottom of the ampoule

(4) Cover the neck of the ampoule with a swab and snap it open

(5) Inspect the solution for glass fragments (discard if present)

(6) Withdraw the required quantity of solution, tilting ampoule if necessary

(7) Replace needle guard and tap syringe to dislodge air bubbles

(8) Expel air

OTHER IMPORTANT NOTES ABOUT INJECTING DRUGS

- Always swab injection site with a cotton wool swab soaked in 70% isopropyl alcohol or antiseptic solution to remove surface debris from skin and hair (exceptions include insulin and vaccinations).
- Before injecting subcutaneous or intramuscular drugs, pull back on syringe plunger. If blood enters the syringe, remove the needle and select a new injection site. This is because the presence of blood in the syringe indicates that a blood vessel has been entered and some agents may cause severe allergic reactions if injected intravenously.

THE WARD

DISPENSING DRUGS

The VN should be able to dispense drugs prescribed by the VS to clients ensuring that all medication is correctly labelled and the dose is correctly calculated.

THE VETERINARY NURSE'S ROLE

- Dispense drugs correctly
- Inform clients of side effects/withdrawal times
- Calculate dosages
- Recognise adverse reactions and drug incompatibilities

POINTS TO REMEMBER WHEN DISPENSING DRUGS

1. Name of the drug?

Drugs are generally referred to by three different names; the *chemical name*, the *generic name* (or nonproprietary) and the *trade name* (or proprietary name).

- *Generic name*: the more concise name given to the specific chemical compound, e.g. amoxicillin
- *Trade name*: unique to each manufacturer for its particular brand of drug, e.g. Clamoxyl™

2. In what form can the drug be dispensed?

Table 8.2 shows in which form drugs may be dispensed.

3. Are there any contraindications?

Every drug comes with a *data sheet*, which contains a large amount of information about that particular drug. The data sheets include the following information:

- *Indications*: are the approved uses for the drug
- *Dose*: that is recommended – the quantities and the frequency of administration
- *Adverse effects*: the effects of the drug *other* than its intended beneficial effect
- *Drug interactions*: highlighting other drugs that may interfere with the effects of the drug in question
- *Contraindications*: conditions when the drug should not be used (e.g. during pregnancy)

Table 8.2 The form in which drugs may be dispensed.

Form of drug	Variations
Tablets Contain the drug in a powdered form, compressed into disks	*Sugar-coated* to make administration easier by hiding the bitter taste of the drug, and help identification. *Capsules* contain the drug in powdered or granular form within a hard gelatin outer case. The gelatin hides a bitter taste and is easier to swallow. *Enteric-coated* tablets contain a special covering over the tablet to prevent it dissolving until it enters the intestine. *Sustained-release* tablets are formulated to release small amounts of drug into the intestine over an extended period of time.
Liquids	*Solutions* contain the dissolved drug in a liquid medium. This mixture does not form a precipitate if left to stand. *Suspensions* contain the drug particles in the liquid, but they are suspended rather than dissolved. This means the drug settles at the bottom of the container if left. It is essential to shake the container to re-suspend the drug thoroughly. *Emulsions* contain a mixture of the drug and liquid fat or oil. *Gels* contain the drug in a semisolid mixture. *Syrups* are solutions of the drug in water and sugar.
Topical applications	*Liniments* contain the drug in an oil-based solution, which are designed to be rubbed onto the skin. *Creams* contain the drug in a semisolid form in oil or fat and water, which are designed to liquefy at body temperatures and spread easily. *Ointments* contain the drug in a semisolid form, which is insoluble in water.
Injectable drugs	Ampoules contain the drug in a small, glass container for single use. Single-dose vials contain enough of the drug for one single administration, e.g. vaccines. Multidose vials are glass bottles of drugs with rubber stoppers. The drug is removed from the vial by inserting the needle through the rubber.

THE WARD

- *Extra-label* or *off-label uses*: of a drug when used in species or for uses other than those intended by the drug's manufacturer

4. What should the drug be put into?
Drug containers
The Council of the Royal Pharmaceutical Society recommends that certain containers be used for the different types of medicines. *Paper envelopes and plastic bags are unacceptable.* Suggested safe containers are listed in Table 8.3.

THE WARD

Table 8.3 Suggested containers for drugs.

Drug type	Container
Topical drugs – shampoo, lotions, eye and ear treatments	Coloured flute bottles
Oral liquids	Plain glass bottles
Blister-pack and sachets	Paper board cartons
Loose tablets or capsules	Plastic, glass or metal containers (preferably child-proof*)
Creams, powders, granules	Wide-mouthed jar

*Normal screw lids may be used with discretion for older clients or those with arthritic hands.

5. What should be written on the label?

The Medicines Act and the Medicine Labelling Regulations state the legal requirements for labelling dispensed drugs. All labels must be legible (preferably computer generated and typed) and indelible.

The following details should be included:

- The owner's name and address
- Date
- Product name and strength
- Total quantity of the product supplied
- Instructions for dosage
- Practice name and address
- 'Keep out of reach of children'
- 'For animal treatment only'

Additional information may include:

- 'For external use only' on labels for products for topical use
- 'WEAR GLOVES when handling drugs'
- 'Give with food'
- 'Give before food'

An example is shown in Fig. 8.1.

6. Which category drug is it?

Dispensing groups

Retail supply of veterinary drugs is restricted to four categories:

- *Prescription Only Medicines* (POM) may be prescribed and dispensed *only* by veterinary surgeons for animals *under their care* (or by a pharmacist on instruction of a veterinary prescription).

For Animal Treatment Only
10 August 1999

For Mrs Sibson's dog Ella
23 Fern Drive, Enniskillen, BT74 5JU

21 x Ampicillin 250mg tablets
Give one tablet three times daily for seven days

Keep All Medicines Out Of Reach Of Children
M Welsh MRCVS
Benmore Small Animal Clinic, 1 Wickham Place, Enniskillen

Fig. 8.1   Example label for dispensed drugs.

- *Controlled Drugs* (CD) are a subcategory of POMs. The rules for supply and storage of these drugs are even more stringent than for general POM medicines.
- *Pharmacy* (P) products may be supplied *only* by veterinary surgeons for animals *under their care* or to the general public by a registered pharmacist.
- *Pharmacy and Merchants List* (PML) products may be supplied by veterinary surgeons for animals under their care, by registered pharmacists or by registered agricultural merchants.
- *General Sales List* (GSL) may be supplied by any retail outlet including supermarkets and pet shops

Drug classifications are different in the Republic of Ireland.

Controlled drugs

Controlled Drugs are regulated by the Misuse of Drugs Act 1971 and the Misuse of Drugs Regulations 1985. These regulations classify such drugs into five schedules (Table 8.4), numbered in decreasing order of severity of control.

7. What precautions should be taken?
Handling of drugs

Safe handling of drugs and knowledge of which ones may pose a health risk to the handler is essential.

The regulations governing the safe handling of drugs are the Health and Safety at Work Act 1974 and the Control of Substances Hazardous to Health (COSHH) Regulations 1999.

Table 8.4 Drug schedules.

Schedule	Example of drugs	Notes
Schedule 1	Includes LSD, cannabis, and other drugs, which are not used medicinally	Possession and supply are prohibited except in accordance with Home Office Authority.
Schedule 2	Includes etorphine, morphine, papaveretum, pethidine, fentanyl (Hypnorm™), diamorphine (heroin), cocaine and amphetamine	Purchase requires a written requisition to the wholesaler or pharmacist by the veterinary surgeon. A bound register of all transactions must be kept. Each different drug should have its own separate section. Registers must be kept for two calendar years after the last entry. Drugs must be kept under safe custody (locked in a secure cabinet).
Schedule 3	Includes buprenorphine (Vetergesic™), pentobarbitone, phenobarbitone and temazepam	These drugs should be locked in a secure cabinet and invoices should be kept for two years.
Schedule 4	Includes butorphanol	Do not need to be locked up.
Schedule 5	Includes preparations such as some of the codeine products (codeine cough linctus and kaolin and morphine suspension).	Invoices should be kept for two years.

Every veterinary practice must have produced a COSHH assessment sheet for *all* substances that staff may come into contact with. This document should:

- Identify the potential risk to handlers
- State the precautions handlers should take to avoid exposure
- List the steps to take in the event of accidental exposure

General rules for safe handling of drugs

- The Health and Safety Regulations state that it is the responsibility of *each individual* to take care of their own health. This means that VNs should take safety into their own hands, not rely on being told by others in the workplace.
- Wear gloves when handling *all* drugs (many capsules and tablets can be safely handled without gloves, however, it is good practice to wear gloves when handling all types of medicine).
- Use a triangular tablet counter when counting tablets to reduce contact of drugs.

- Wear face masks and eye goggles when handling powders and/or aerosol sprays.
- Dispose of used needles and syringes immediately after use. Dispose of contaminated packages and bottles appropriately.
- Keep all food and drink away from the pharmacy and wash hands before eating, drinking or smoking.
- Thoroughly clean surfaces after working with drugs in that area.

LEGAL ASPECTS OF MEDICINES AND PRESCRIBING

The following regulations and acts are concerned with how veterinary practices buy, sell, store, prescribe drugs and the safety issues concerned.

- The Medicines Act 1968 (Dealing with Distribution Categories)
- The Medicines (Restrictions on the Administration of Veterinary Medicinal Products) Regulations 1994
- The Misuse of Drugs Act 1971 (see section above on Controlled drugs)
- The Misuse of Drugs Regulations 1985 (see section above on Controlled drugs)
- The Health and Safety at Work Act 1974
- The Control of Substances Hazardous to Health Regulations 1999

THE WARD

CHAPTER 9

PREPARATION AND ADMINISTRATION OF AN ENEMA

INTRODUCTION

Enema: a liquid introduced into the rectum.

Indications

- To empty the rectum
- To relieve constipation or impaction
- Prior to surgery/radiography/colonoscopy
- To administer radiographic contrast media
- To irrigate the colon in some poisoning cases

Table 9.1 indicates the solutions that may be used, and the quantities to give.

Table 9.1 Solutions and quantities to give.

Solution	Quantity	General points
Warm water	Cat 5–10 ml/kg Small–medium dog 20–30 ml/kg Large dog 30–40 ml/kg Repeat ever 20–30 minutes if necessary	Cheap Easy to use Nonirritant
Liquid paraffin	5–10 ml/kg every 1–2 hours	Cheap and effective but very messy
Contrast medium – barium sulphate	7–14 ml/kg	Radiographic contrast media
Proprietary agent	As directed by manufacturers	e.g. Microlax™
Phosphate enemas	As directed by manufacturers	Do not use for small dogs and cats because this preparation may cause hypocalcaemia and collapse
Saline	1–2 ml/kg Do not repeat for up to 12 hours	Use with care in small dogs and cats

EQUIPMENT

- Enema solution (warmed)
- Gloves
- Plastic apron
- Lubricant
- Syringe
- Soft rubber tube or Higginson's syringe
- Funnel or large catheter tip syringe
- Jug for containing and pouring enema solution

TECHNIQUE

(1) Gather all equipment together
(2) If possible, take the animal to an outdoor exercise run/ kennel or stand in wash basin or bathtub
(3) Provide litter tray for cats
(4) Assistant restrain animal (standing position)
(5) Put on gloves
(6) Place enema solution in to jug
(7) Lubricate the nozzle of enema tubing and anal ring
(8) Hold tail up and away and insert tube gently into the anus
(9) Gently advance the tube, rotating slightly and moving the tube back and forth to advance the tube into the rectum
(10) Hold the free end of the tube as high as it will allow and attach funnel or syringe
(11) Pour enema solution into the tube (stand to one side)
(12) Remove the tube after administering required amount of fluid
(13) Leave animal to evacuate rectum
(14) Write time of administration on patient's records

ADDITIONAL NOTES

- A gloved, lubricated finger may be inserted into the rectum to break up hard faeces
- Do not work on constipated animals for more than 20 minutes at any one time. Wait for an hour and repeat the procedure

- Severe impaction may take multiple administrations over several days or a general anaesthetic and manual evacuation
- Cats may require sedation prior to enema administration; use small amounts with low pressure

Strong soap solutions, hydrogen peroxide and hot water enemas irritate the mucosa and should not be used.

CHAPTER 10

URINARY CATHETERISATION

Urinary catheterisation requires passing a catheter into the bladder via the urethra. There is a risk of iatrogenic trauma and infection and so the VN must ensure that the correct and aseptic technique is used.

Indications for urinary catheterisation:

1. Obtain sterile sample

- When the patient will not urinate
- For bacteria culture and sensitivity tests – (free catch may be contaminated)

2. To empty the bladder

- Before abdominal, vaginal or urethral surgery
- Before radiography – pneumocystogram
- To relieve urine retention

3. Introduce contrast media

- For radiographic procedures – bladder investigation or to check the patency of the urethra

4. Maintain constant and controlled bladder drainage

- In recumbent or comatose patients to prevent soiling
- After bladder surgery to prevent tension on suture line

5. Hydropropulsion methods

- Use of water pressure to dislodge particles in the urethra

6. Maintain patent urethra

- Cats with feline urological syndrome (allows drainage whilst treatment is initiated and to flush the bladder with antibiotics)
- To relieve dysuria or anuria in the nonsurgical patient

7. Monitor urine output

- Check kidney function
- During intensive care
- After renal surgery to ensure adequate production of urine (1–2 ml/kg/hour)

8. Introduction of drugs

- Antibiotics, etc.

COMPLICATIONS WITH CATHETERISATION

INFECTION

Urinary tract infection (UTI) may occur easily if the bacterium in the urethra is pushed into the bladder. The risk of infection is increased when:

- The tract is traumatised
- Aseptic technique not used
- Presence of vaginal or preputial discharge
- Indwelling catheters used
- The patient is immunosuppressed and therefore susceptible to infection
- Repeated catheterisation

TRAUMA

- Some epithelial damage may occur in male dogs as the catheter is passed around the ischial curve
- Force applied during catheterisation
- Inadequate lubrication of the catheter

PATIENT RESISTANCE

- This is an uncomfortable procedure, especially in bitches or queens
- May be necessary to sedate or anaesthetise the animal

BLOCKAGE

- May be due to small calculi blocking the catheter – flush with sterile saline or water

PATIENT INTERFERENCE

- Patients are likely to remove indwelling catheters – use Elizabethan collar and ensure catheter is sutured adequately

TYPES OF URINARY CATHETERS

Catheters come in a variety of shapes, sizes and materials (see Tables 10.1 and 10.2). Catheters are designed for single use only, however, they may be cleaned thoroughly and sterilised by ethylene oxide provided that there is no damage to the catheter.

ADDITIONAL EQUIPMENT REQUIRED FOR CATHETERISATION

1. SPECULUM

- Metal instruments used to enable visualisation of the urethral orifice
- Auroscopes may be adapted also for this use
- Must be sterile

2. LIGHT SOURCE

- Pen torch/head light

3. STYLET

- To aid the use of the more flexible catheters (e.g. Foley)
- Usually made of metal, easily sterilised.

Table 10.1 Choosing a urinary catheter.

Animal	Appropriate size of catheter	Suitable catheter for animal	Sizes available	Catheter material
Male or female cat	3–4 French gauge 3–4 FG	Tom cat catheter Jackson catheter	3 and 4 FG	Nylon Nylon
Male dog				
< 5 kg	3.5–5 FG	Dog catheter	6–10 FG	Nylon
5–23 kg	8 FG			(polyamide)
> 23 kg	10–12 FG			
Female dog				
< 5 kg	5 FG	Tieman's	8–12 FG	PVC
5–23 kg	8 FG	Foley	8–16 FG	Latex
> 23 kg	10–14 FG	Metal	Various	Brass plated

Table 10.2 Types of urinary catheters.

Bitch	Dog	Cat
Foley Latex, inflatable balloon helps to maintain the position of the catheter in the bladder. Inflate with appropriate amount of air/water. Deflate before removal. Single use/indwelling May require metal stylet Petroleum-based lubricants damage the latex Size range 8–16 French Gauge *Tiemans* PVC, single use catheters Primarily designed for human males! Curved tip useful for locating urethra but length too long Size range 8–12 FG *Metal (Dowe's) catheter* Plated brass Not used now as can be too rigid and traumatic Various sizes available	Made from flexible nylon May be used as indwelling catheters using 'butterfly' tapes to suture to the skin Can be used also as bitch catheters Size range 6–10 FG	Conventional Nylon Single use Smaller version of dog catheters Size range 3 and 4 FG Jackson Indwelling 'tom cat' catheters Nylon with additional metal stylet and plastic flange to suture to the prepuce Size range 3 and 4 FG

4. SYRINGE

- For inflating/deflating Foley balloon

5. BUNGS AND SPIGOTS

- To block the distal free end of the catheter if left as an indwelling catheter

6. THREE-WAY TAP

- Useful when draining the bladder

7. URINE COLLECTION BAGS

- Prepacked and sterile for single use only
- One way valve ensures no urine can track back
- Empty drip bags with giving sets may also be used

GENERAL POINTS FOR METHODS OF URINARY CATHETERISATION

ASEPTIC TECHNIQUE

- Is important to ensure no infection occurs
- Use sterile surgical gloves when digital catheterisation is performed

RESTRAINT

- Physical, or
- Chemical restraint (sedation or general anaesthetic may be necessary)

PREPARE EQUIPMENT

- Ensure all equipment is ready before restraining the patient

LUBRICATION

- KY jelly™ most commonly used, will not damage latex
- 2% lignocaine hydrochloride gel (Xylocaine™) may be used – helps desensitise the prepuce or vestibule

CLEANING OF PATIENT

- Clip and clean around external genitalia if necessary
- Remove discharges or dirt

GLOVES

- Nonsterile gloves adequate (health and safety reasons)

LENGTH OF CATHETER

- Do not insert an over-long catheter too far – it can bend, kink, re-enter the bladder or damage the bladder wall

TECHNIQUES

CATHETERISATION OF MALE DOGS

(1) Collect equipment

(2) Assistant to restrain dog in lateral recumbency and hold the upper portion of the hindlimb away from the site of operation

(3) Estimate the length of catheter to be inserted (without jeopardising asepsis)

(4) Clip the hair at the end of the prepuce if the dog is long haired

(5) Gently cleanse the prepuce with surgical scrub

(6) Rinse well (soap may cause the urine sample to appear cloudy and inhibit micro-organism growth if being sent for culture)

(7) Wash hands and wear gloves

(8) Another assistant opens external catheter package to enable operator to take sterile inner pack

(9) Cut the end off the catheter package and cut a further 'feeder' section approximately 2.5 cm long (see Fig. 10.1)

(10) Expose just the tip of the catheter and apply sterile lubricant (2% lignocaine hydrochloride gel)

(11) Retract the prepuce to expose the penis

(12) Use the other hand to pass the catheter into the urethral opening

(13) Continue feeding the catheter along the urethra gently (it should pass easily – if this is not the case, re-evaluate the size of the catheter)

(14) When the catheter reaches the ischial arch, gently rotate the catheter and continue to push with steady pressure

(15) Once the catheter is in the bladder, urine should begin to flow into the package

(16) Discard the first few millilitres and collect 6–10 ml in a sterile syringe if required for analysis

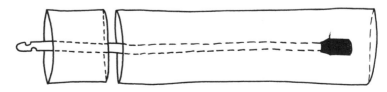

Fig. 10.1   Method for aseptically handling the catheter.

Never twist the catheter harshly whilst in the urethra as this can cause trauma and never apply digital pressure to the bladder when the catheter is in place because the catheter may traumatise the bladder.

CATHETERISATION OF FEMALE DOGS

(1) Collect equipment
(2) Assistant to restrain dog in standing position and hold the tail to one side, away from the site of operation (some operators prefer the dog to be in lateral recumbency)
(3) Estimate the length of catheter to be inserted (without jeopardising asepsis)
(4) Clip the hair from around the vulva if the dog is long haired
(5) Gently cleanse the lips of the vulva with surgical scrub
(6) Wash hands and wear gloves
(7) Another assistant opens external catheter package to enable operator to take sterile inner pack and leaves it to one side so that it can be used to rest the catheter
(8) Open the inner pack and apply sterile lubricant to the tip of the catheter
(9) Rest the catheter on the opened sterile pack
(10) Lubricate the sterile speculum (vaginoscope, otoscope or nasal speculum can be used)
(11) Using one hand, insert the speculum into the vagina and direct the tip first dorsally, then cranially (to avoid the clitoral fossa)
(12) Visually locate the urethral orifice on the ventral floor of the vagina approximately 3–5 cm inside the vagina
(13) Use the other hand to pass the catheter into the urethral opening
(14) Withdraw the speculum, taking care not to dislodge the catheter tip
(15) Continue feeding the catheter along the urethra gently (it should pass easily – if this is not the case, re-evaluate the size of the catheter or use a stylet with Foley catheter)
(16) Once the catheter is in the bladder, urine should begin to flow
(17) Discard the first few millilitres and collect 6–10 ml in a sterile syringe if required for analysis

THE WARD

Some people prefer not to use a speculum when catheterising bitches. Instead they locate the urethral opening manually. This technique takes more practice initially but is less awkward than trying to manage the speculum and catheter at the same time. Using a gloved, lubricated finger, insert into the vagina dorsally and then cranially for approximately 3 cm. Gently palpate the vestibular floor to feel for the urethral papilla, which feels like a soft, round mass 0.5–1 cm in diameter. (This is just cranial to a slight depression in the vaginal floor.)

Placing the finger on top of the papilla the other hand passes the catheter beneath the papilla down into the urethra. (If the catheter can be felt passing directly underneath the finger, it is misdirected and should be redirected correctly.)

CATHETERISATION OF MALE CATS

General anaesthesia or sedation is usually required for urinary catheterisation of the male cat.

(1) Collect equipment
(2) Assistant to restrain cat in dorsal recumbency and hold the hindlimbs cranially away from the site of operation
(3) Estimate the length of catheter to be inserted (without jeopardising asepsis)
(4) Gently cleanse the prepuce with surgical scrub
(5) Wash hands and wear gloves
(6) Another assistant opens external catheter package to enable operator to take sterile inner pack
(7) Cut the end off the catheter package and cut a further 'feeder' section approximately 2.5 cm long
(8) Expose just the tip of the catheter and apply sterile lubricant
(9) Retract the prepuce to expose the penis and gently put traction on the penis in a caudal direction to help straighten the penile flexure
(10) Use the other hand to pass the catheter into the urethral opening (keeping the catheter parallel to the spine)
(11) Continue feeding the catheter along the urethra gently (it should pass easily – if this is not the case, re-evaluate the size of the catheter)
(12) Once the catheter is in the bladder, urine should begin to flow into the package
(13) Discard the first few millilitres and collect 6–10 ml in a sterile syringe if required for analysis

Never twist the catheter harshly whilst in the urethra as this can cause trauma and never apply digital pressure to the bladder when the catheter is in place because the catheter may traumatise the bladder.

CATHETERISATION OF FEMALE CATS

Sedation or general anaesthesia is required to perform urinary catheterisation of the female cat. It is a difficult procedure and one that is rarely carried out.

(1) Collect equipment
(2) Assistant to restrain cat in lateral recumbency and hold the tail to one side away from the site of operation
(3) Estimate the length of catheter to be inserted (without jeopardising asepsis)
(4) Gently cleanse around the vulva with surgical scrub
(5) Rinse
(6) Wash hands and wear gloves
(7) Another assistant opens external catheter package to enable operator to take sterile inner pack
(8) Expose just the tip of the catheter and apply sterile lubricant
(9) With one hand insert a small lubricated sterile speculum into the vagina and locate the urethral orifice on the vestibular floor
(10) With the other hand, pass the catheter into the urethral orifice
(11) Continue feeding the catheter along the urethra gently
(12) Once the catheter is in the bladder, urine should begin to flow into the package
(13) Discard the first few millilitres and collect 6–10 ml in a sterile syringe if required for analysis

FURTHER READING

Anderson, R.E. (1991) *Practical Animal Handling*. Pergamon, Oxford.

Thorne, C. (ed) (1992) *The Waltham Book of Dog & Cat Behaviour*. Pergamon, Oxford.

THE WARD

SECTION 2
THEATRE PRACTICE

CHAPTER 11

AN INTRODUCTION TO THEATRE MANAGEMENT

THE HISTORICAL DEVELOPMENT OF THEATRE PRACTICE AND ASEPTIC TECHNIQUE

Until the nineteenth century, surgery was rarely carried out because of the extremely high incidence of postoperative infection. It was not until the mid-1800s that people realised that scrupulous cleaning of hands by operating personnel caused a significant drop in postoperative mortality. The strict theatre protocols that are in place today; the wearing of gowns, gloves, hats and masks, etc., is as a direct result of realising that an aseptic technique is required to help prevent postoperative infection.

THEATRE MANAGEMENT

It is the job of the VN to manage the theatre suite. Many of the larger clinics and teaching hospitals employ a nurse to work specifically in this area because they identify that theatre efficiency can be maximised by ensuring that a highly qualified and specialised person is involved with the day-to-day running of the area. In terms of general practice, the veterinary nurse can use his or her expertise to raise standards of hygiene and sanitation in the theatre and organise the area and other veterinary colleagues to maximise operating room order and efficiency.

RESPONSIBILITIES INCLUDE

- Maintaining theatre hygiene
- Cleaning surgical equipment
- Sterilising equipment
- Maintaining surgical instruments

Table 11.1   Ideal operating theatre design.

Room	Equipment required
Theatre. Should be isolated, convenient with no through-traffic. It should contain only basic equipment and no more. Clutter should be cleared-out, or at the very least put away into cupboards. Adequate lighting, easy to clean walls and floors. Heating 21°C. Positive pressure ventilation with bacterial filters.	Adjustable operating table Anaesthetic machine Piped gases (if available) Scavenging equipment 'Kick-about' waste bowls X-ray viewing screen (flush with wall) Instrument trolley (Mayo, two-tier, over-table type) Clock
Preparation room. This is where the animal is anaesthetised, clipped and prepared for surgery. Dirty procedures such as dental surgery and abscess lancing should be carried out here to reduce contamination of theatre.	Preparation table with built in sink Anaesthetic machine and circuits Clippers (on reel from wall or ceiling) Vacuum cleaner Skin preparation solutions Weighing scales Anaesthetic drugs and emergency box
Scrub room. This is where the surgical team scrub, gown and glove. It should be next to theatre but not in same room (moist conditions encourage bacteria).	Stainless steel scrub sinks Elbow, knee or foot operated hot and cold water Antiseptic skin scrub solutions and sterile brushes located above sinks Sterile gowns and gloves (away from splash area)
Sterile store. If stored in closed cabinets the packs will remain sterile for longer than if left out on open shelves. Kits and instruments may be kept in the theatre in closed cabinets so that they are close to hand.	All sterile equipment and kits Any additional non-routine equipment Disposable sterile items
Instrument preparation and sterilisation room. Situated away from the theatre, the dirty instruments and drapes can be brought here to be washed and resterilised.	Sink(s) Washing machine/dryer Ultrasonic cleaners Instrument lubrication Sterilising units (autoclave, hot air oven) Adequate bench space for preparing and packing kits Stock of sterilising pouches, tape, indicators, etc. Clinical waste bins
Recovery and treatment room. This should be somewhere quiet and warm where the animals can recover safely whilst being constantly monitored.	Recovery cages (all sizes) Monitoring equipment Crash trolley with emergency drugs and equipment Oxygen administering equipment Intravenous fluids (in warming cabinet) Heat pads, waterbeds and incubator Bedding supplies, etc.

- Surgical preparation of the patient
- Intraoperative patient care
- Assisting during surgical procedures
- Performing minor surgical procedures (according to amendment to the Veterinary Surgeons Act in 1991)

THE OPERATING ROOM AND ENVIRONMENT

In an ideal situation, the operating room and environment should be spacious, purpose built and used specifically for the purpose of operating and nothing else. Table 11.1 identifies aspects of theatre design that are the ideal and explains why.

METHODS OF PREVENTING INFECTION IN THEATRE

- Routinely disinfect theatres
- Restrict movement through the theatre area
- No through-traffic
- Surgeons to scrub and glove effectively
- Check sterilisation methods regularly
- Every one in theatre to wear clean scrub suits and theatre shoes
- Use appropriate order for surgical procedures, i.e. clean operations before dirty operations (e.g. orthopaedic operations before dental operations, bitch spay before gastrointestinal surgery)
- Ensure adequate clipped area on the patient
- Aseptic operative technique
- Keep surgical time as short as possible

CHAPTER 12

PREPARATION OF THE THEATRE FOR SURGERY

Maintenance of asepsis in theatre is very important, therefore cleaning protocols should be adhered to.

PROCEDURE

EVERY DAY BEFORE THE SURGICAL SESSION

- Damp-dust the operating room with disinfectant (all surfaces and equipment)
- Check the theatre list and set up equipment ready for use
- Collect all instruments that may be required for the operation
- Ensure the anaesthetic machine and circuits are working

BETWEEN SURGICAL CASES

- Remove and clean instruments and equipment
- Remove all waste materials (tissues, swabs, empty packets)
- Clean and disinfect 'kick-about' bowl
- Clean and disinfect operating table and instrument trolley
- Clean gross dirt (blood, etc.) from floor
- Set up for next operation

AFTER SURGICAL SESSION

- Remove all instruments and equipment for cleaning and sterilising
- Clean and disinfect all surfaces, lights, equipment and walls

- Disinfect an area of the floor so that the equipment may be rolled on to this spot whilst the rest of the floor is cleaned
- Restock for next session
- It is useful to obtain swabs for bacteriology from the operating room environment periodically

CLEANING EQUIPMENT AND SUPPLIES

Wet-vacuums are preferable to mops when washing floors. They can be used with disinfectant. Mops are a potential source of infection. They must be rinsed thoroughly after each use, and then soaked in disinfectant for 30 minutes before standing on end to dry.

Disposable gloves should be worn when cleaning theatre and equipment as they help to prevent infection and protect against irritant/harmful effects of some cleaning and disinfectant products, as well as potential zoonoses.

Cloths and sponges should preferably be disposable to minimise contamination, otherwise, launder and dry daily.

CHAPTER 13

PREPARATION OF THE SURGICAL TEAM

One of the possible contaminants in the theatre is the personnel involved with the surgery. Changing into theatre clothing and scrupulous cleaning of the hands help reduce the risk. Table 13.1 lists the types of clothing necessary.

THE SURGICAL SCRUB

OBJECTIVES

- Mechanical removal of gross dirt
- Reduction of transient micro-organisms
- Reduction of residual micro-organisms
- Prolonged depressant effect on resident microflora

The entire scrub should last between 5 and 7 minutes.

PROCEDURE

(1) Remove jewellery
(2) Cut nails short
(3) Regulate water temperature

Table 13.1 Theatre clothing.

Theatre clothing	
Clothing	Scrub suit (two-piece or dress), use clean pair every day
Footwear	Antistatic, only worn in theatre, clean regularly
Hats	Cloth or disposable, must contain all hair
Masks	Must cover mouth and nose
	Do not reduce environmental contamination
	Efficiency is reduced when moist (effective for first 20 minutes only)
Sterile gowns	Cloth or disposable

(4) Wash arms and hands working up a good lather

(5) Rinse hands keeping them above the elbows

(6) Using sterile scrub brush, scrub arms and hands

(7) Use ten strokes on each surface

(8) Work in a specific order – left hand, left arm, right hand, right arm, etc.

(9) Rinse, repeat

(10) Wash again with solution

(11) Rinse and drain

CHOOSING A SKIN ANTISEPTIC

Types of skin antiseptic are shown in Table 13.2.

Table 13.2 Skin antiseptics.

Chemical	Other name	Trade name	Action
Chlorhexidine	Chlorhexidine gluconate 4%	Dinex scrub Vetasept	Reasonably effective against many bacteria
	Chlorhexidine gluconate	Hibiscrub	Not as effective as povidone-iodine at killing fungi
	Chlorhexidine acetate 0.1%	Nolvadent	Effective against many viruses
	Chlorhexidine acetate	Nolvasan	Medium activity (longer than povidone-iodine
	Chlorhexidine gluconate cetrimide	Savlon	Chemically active for long time (6 hours)
			Daily use leads to lowered skin bacteria counts over time
			Not affected by organic matter
			Little skin irritation
			Irritant to mucous membranes
Iodine/ iodophors	Povidone-iodine	Pevidine	Effective against wide range of bacteria, viruses and fungi
			Some activity against spores
			Not easily inactivated by organic matter
			Rapid initial activity time (2 minutes)
			Shorter activity time than chlorhexidine
			Allergic effects often seen
Alcohols	Usually used in combination with chlorhexidine as hand rubs	Vetasept Chlorhexidine Clear Vetasept Hand Rub	Ineffective against bacterial spores

GOWNING AND GLOVING

After the scrub procedure is completed, the hands are dried using a sterile towel. A sterile gown is then put on taking care not to touch the outside of the gown. The sterile gloves are then put on using the 'open', 'closed' or 'plunge' method.

GOWNING

The gown should be packed and sterilised so that the inside of the gown is outermost with the neck of the gown on top.

Procedure

(1)   Grasp the gown neck. Moving away from any surfaces allow the gown to unravel taking care not to allow the gown to touch the floor.

(2)   Slide each arm into the sleeves alternately, touching only the inside of the gown.

(3)   If an open gloving technique is used the cuffs should be at wrist level, if a closed technique is used then the hands should remain inside the sleeves.

(4)   The assistant should now stand behind the gowned person to adjust the gown over the shoulders holding the neck ties and only touching the inside of the gown if necessary. The neck ties are then tied.

(5)   If the gown has front ties, the gowned person should lean forward and grasp the ties holding them out to the sides.

(6)   The assistant can then grab the ends of the ties and tie them behind the gowned person.

(7)   Self-tying gowns (usually the disposable kind) have the waist ties incorporated into a piece of card on the front of the gown.

(8)   The assistant takes hold of the card not touching the ties whilst the gowned person releases one tie from the card and turns around. This action causes the tie to wrap around the waist of the gowned person so that he or she can then tie the two ties together at the waist, thereby securing the gown.

GLOVING

The sterile gloves are put on immediately after putting on the gown.

Procedure
1. Plunge method
The easiest of all methods. A scrubbed and gloved assistant holds the gloves open for the surgeon to 'plunge' their hand straight into the glove. Ensure the assistant knows their left from their right!

2. Open method

(1)   Remember – only touch the inside of the gloves.
(2)   The inner glove packet is opened.
(3)   Pick up the cuff of the right glove with the left hand and place the right hand into the glove.
(4)   As the hand is placed into the glove use the thumb to catch the edge of the cuff – this will help when putting the other glove on.
(5)   Using the right partially gloved hand, slide the gloved fingers under the cuff of the left glove.
(6)   Use the right thumb to hold the cuff and slide the left hand into the left glove. At the same time pull the folded-over edge of the cuff over the sleeve on the left arm pulling the glove on fully.
(7)   The gloved fingers of the left hand can now be hooked under the cuff on the right glove and the glove is pulled on fully over the sleeve on the right arm.
(8)   Adjust the gloves carefully so that they fit comfortably.

3. Closed gloving
Closed gloving must be carried out on a sterile surface and the hands are retained within the sleeves of the gown.

(1)   Open the inner glove packet on a sterile drape.
(2)   Grasp the cuff of the right glove with the right fingers and thumb which is still covered by the gown sleeve. The fingers of the glove should lie along the wrist pointing towards the body with the thumb of the glove closest to the wrist.

THEATRE PRACTICE

(3) With the left hand pull the cuff over the right hand whilst thrusting the right hand into the glove. Ensure the cuff of the glove covers all of the cuff of the sleeve.

(4) Repeat the same procedure with the left glove.

(5) Pick up the left glove with the fingers and thumb of the left hand, which is still covered by the sleeve of the gown.

(6) Grasp the cuff of the glove with the right hand pulling it over the left hand whilst thrusting the left hand into the glove.

(7) Once both gloves are on then slight adjustments for comfort may be made.

After gloving, the hands should be clasped together above the waist and in front of the chest to reduce chances of contamination.

The area from neck to waist at the front of the scrubbed person including the arms and gloved hands is considered sterile.

CHAPTER 14

PREPARATION OF THE PATIENT FOR THEATRE

Preparation of any surgical patient begins as soon as the animal arrives at the hospital. The VN may be responsible for many of the tasks carried out during the patient's stay at the hospital and it is essential that he or she has a thorough knowledge of the techniques employed and the pertinence of particular procedures to each surgical case.

ADMISSION TO THE HOSPITAL

An admissions check list (this can be incorporated into the consent form) can be used to verify the patient's identity and proposed surgical procedure; confirm that food and water have been withheld for the required length of time and have space for the owner's signature for consent to treatment and surgery. An estimate of the total cost of treatment can also be included.

A general clinical examination and weight check should be performed and the results recorded. Any abnormalities should be reported to the VS. The patient may be exercised prior to admittance to allow urination and defecation.

A note should be made of previous and current medication treatments (some medications may affect anaesthetic protocols or medication regimes). It may be useful in some cases to determine if the animal has had a blood transfusion in the past, as subsequent transfusion will require cross-matching.

GENERAL PREPARATION

- Bath (day before)
- Food withheld for 12 hours (adult cats and dogs)
- Withhold water 2–3 hours prior to surgery (unless suffering from renal disease)

- Allow urination/defecation
- Enema – if required
- Placement of intravenous catheter (facilitates smoother induction, reduces risk of accidental perivascular injection, allows intravenous fluid administration and ensures a route for drugs in the event of an anaesthetic emergency)

PREMEDICATION

Pre-anaesthetic medication is frequently administered prior to induction of general anaesthesia for a number of reasons.

- To calm and control the patient
- To provide analgesia throughout surgery
- To reduce the amount of anaesthetic induction and maintenance agent required
- To produce a smooth induction of anaesthetic
- To reduce some of the unwanted side-effects of some anaesthetic agents
- To ensure a smoother recovery from anaesthesia

HAIR REMOVAL

- Removal of fur should be carried out in a separate room to the operating theatre.
- Use a number 40 Oster clipper blade.
- For delicate areas and around the eye, it is useful to use small clippers with a narrower blade. The use of a depilatory or razor is not recommended for use in animals because of their irritant effect on the skin.
- As a general guide, the clipped area should radiate approximately 10 cm around the surgical incision.
- The blade of the clippers should be kept flat against the skin to prevent excessive trauma to the skin.
- Spray blades frequently with a commercial blade coolant and lubricant to help prevent excoriation or clipper burns.
- The blades must be sharp and free of broken teeth to prevent skin abrasions.
- A sterile water soluble gel can be applied to any pre-existing open wounds or on to the surface of the eye as protection (unless intra-ocular surgery is being performed). Fine loose

hairs can then be washed away easily during the cleaning stage.

- Loose fur can be removed from the skin, body and surrounding area by vacuuming or by using sticky tape around delicate areas.

PATIENT POSITIONING

- The VS will often decide how he or she will want the patient positioned, however, for many procedures there will be a standard position and the VN should be familiar with these.
- Positioning should only be carried out after the anaesthetic has been stabilised.
- Take care not to compromise circulatory or respiratory function.
- Placing the animal on a thermostatically controlled hot water bed or electric blanket will help to prevent hypothermia during surgery. Care must be taken with some heated pads, which may cause severe burning.
- When performing surgery on a limb, cover the distal part of the leg with a conforming bandage and suspend the leg from a drip stand. This will aid in the cleaning procedure and give the surgeon full access to drape the limb. See Fig. 14.1.

SKIN DISINFECTION

There are many solutions available for use on skin, it is important to select a solution with a detergent agent to remove gross dirt and grease and which also contains an antimicrobial agent effective against a wide range of micro-organisms. The solution must remain active in the presence of organic matter, should not cause any skin irritation and have a long residual effect. Commonly, chlorhexidine or povidone-iodine solutions are used for veterinary purposes.

- Skin antiseptics
- Povidone-iodine
- Chlorhexidine
- Alcohol

THEATRE PRACTICE

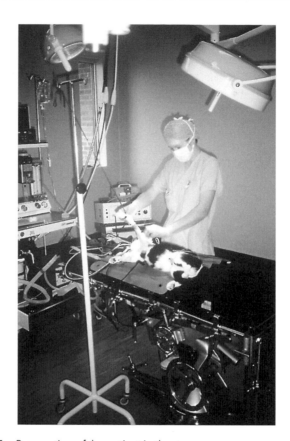

Fig. 14.1 Preparation of the patient in theatre.

Procedure

(1) Wear gloves (reduces bacterial numbers)
(2) Clean gross dirt from the site first
(3) Use a clean swab each time
(4) Start at the incision site and work outwards to the edge taking care not to swab from contaminated area to clean area
(5) Continue until no more obvious dirt is removed by the swab
(6) Avoid excessive scrubbing as this will cause skin irritation
(7) Lather the area well but avoid soaking the animal or it will get cold
(8) Flatten hair around the edges by damping it down
(9) Alcohol may be used after scrub solution to remove the lather and additional antisepsis (do not use on open

wounds, mucous membranes or small mammals susceptible to hypothermia)

(10) A final solution of povidone-iodine may then be used on the area using sterile swabs and Cheatle forceps

(11) The discoloration of the skin indicates where the surgical site has been prepared for draping and the solution provides continued bactericidal activity

Chlorhexidine is active against a wide range of bacteria and many fungi. It does not become deactivated when exposed to organic matter or alcohol and it has been shown to produce a 99% bacterial kill rate 30 seconds after application. Chlorhexidine has longer residual activity than povidone-iodine. Chlorhexidine is irritant to the cornea and should not be used around the eyes; instead, a 2% solution of povidone-iodine may be used followed by a sterile saline flush.

Povidone-iodine continues its bactericidal activity by the release of free iodine as it dries and the colour fades. As with chlorhexidine, it is effective against a wide range of bacteria and fungi. Its effectiveness is reduced by the presence of organic material (e.g. blood and fat) and is therefore best left as a final spray or paint solution after the initial preparation with chlorhexidine and isopropyl alcohol.

Isopropyl alcohol is effective against a wide range of gram-negative organisms and some fungal spores. It is useful to apply isopropyl alcohol after scrubbing the skin because is removes the lather produced by the scrub solution and has a drying effect on the skin. Isopropyl alcohol should not be used on mucous membranes or on open wounds because it causes tissue necrosis.

Care must be taken to avoid wetting the patient too much during the preparation stage to reduce the risk of hypothermia. The evaporation effect of applying isopropyl alcohol also creates a cooling effect and it is probably better to avoid using it in very small or neonatal animals.

DRAPING THE PATIENT

Drapes are one of the main barriers against contamination during surgery and should be large enough to cover the patient and the whole operating table. Drapes can be made of cotton, paper or plastic. Cotton drapes have the advantage of being reusable and therefore cost effective, they conform well to the patient. However, their main disadvantage is that when wet, they become a carrier for bacterial strike-through from the patient to the surgeon. Water repellent paper drapes and plastic drapes reduce the risk of moisture contamination but are more expensive. Table 14.1 lists the advantages and disadvantages of different types of drapes.

PROCEDURE

(1) The drapes are removed from their sterile packaging by a scrubbed assistant or the surgeon and unfolded away from any contaminating surfaces.

(2) Once opened, one edge should be folded over by about 10 cm to create an area of double thickness.

(3) The first drape is placed between the surgeon and the operating table over the animal to prevent any contamination of the surgeon from the table or patient.

(4) Once placed, the drapes should not be moved towards the incision site to avoid bringing contaminants towards the site.

(5) The remaining drapes are positioned and then secured to the patient using towel clamps, see Fig. 14.2.

(6) Additional draping can be utilised to provide a second protective layer between the patient and surgeon.

(7) Adhesive plastic drapes may be utilised, these are placed directly onto the skin and the surgical incision is then made through this layer. They provide a waterproof barrier and are quick to apply, however, the presence of stubble and moisture on the skin surface prevents them sticking well.

The 'towelling-in' method of skin draping involves suturing disposable paper drapes to the skin edges after the initial skin

Table 14.1 Comparison of disposable and nondisposable drapes.

Type of drapes	Advantages	Disadvantages
Disposable drapes	Labour saving No laundering Some are presterilised More water repellent	Expensive Not as conforming or as easy to handle
Cotton drapes	Cheaper Conforming Easier to handle	Bacterial strike-through if wet Time consuming – washing, folding and sterilisation

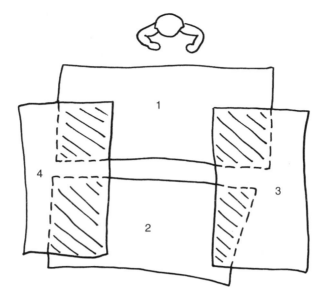

Fig. 14.2 Draping the patient.

incision is made. Whilst time-consuming, this provides an effective barrier against bacteria by completely isolating the surgical site from the surrounding skin surface.

THEATRE PRACTICE

CHAPTER 15

ASSISTING DURING SURGERY

INTRA-OPERATIVE CARE – THE SCRUB NURSE

The VN is an important member of the surgical team and must be fully competent in assisting the VS during surgical procedures.

The main tasks of the scrub nurse during a surgical procedure include:

- Assisting the surgeon (without distracting or slowing the surgeon down)
- Assisting with the control of haemorrhage
- Anticipating the surgeon's needs
- Keeping the instrument trolley tidy
- Handling body tissues and keeping them moist
- Cutting sutures correctly

It is important to note the following points when assisting with surgery.

(1) When assisting during a surgical procedure, take care not to block the surgeon's view of the operating field or create shadows by standing in the way of light sources.
(2) Know all the names of the instruments that are being used during each procedure and anticipate what instrument will be required next.
(3) Pass the instrument to the surgeon so that the handle is placed into their hand: take particular care when passing scalpel blades and sharp instruments.
(4) Keep the instrument trolley in order. At the start of surgery, arrange instruments on the trolley in the anticipated order of use (e.g. scalpel handle, scissors, rat tooth forceps …).
(5) Place used, bloody instruments on one side of the trolley and keep them separate from the clean, unused instruments.

(6) Control haemorrhage throughout surgery using gauze swabs as necessary. Anticipate when you will run out of gauze swabs and request more from the theatre nurse.

(7) Count all swabs at the start and end of each procedure. Keep track of the number used to avoid any being accidentally left inside a body cavity. (Yes, it does happen!)

(8) When swabbing haemorrhaging tissues, use a dabbing motion rather than wiping as this can impair clotting and damage delicate tissue.

(9) Control haemorrhage from a vessel by applying pressure with a finger or gauze swab until the surgeon can apply a haemostat (the tips of the clamp trap the severed ends of the vessel). This may be left in place or ligated with suture material.

(10) Pass cautery instrumentation for haemorrhage control to the surgeon if it is available.

(11) Moisten sterile gauze swabs with warm saline and apply to any drying tissues. (Drying can lead to tissue damage).

(12) If suction equipment is available and necessary (e.g. during abdominal lavage or severe haemorrhage) use an appropriate suction tip and try to avoid adhering the end of the tip to the surrounding soft tissues.

(13) Handle all tissues and organs gently; aggressive manipulation of these can cause trauma, bruising and haemorrhage.

(14) Do not replace bloody swabs or discarded tissue matter onto the trolley, drop them into the kick bin.

(15) Cut sutures to the required length after a knot has been tied. Use blunt ended scissors and avoid inadvertently nipping any surrounding tissues.

(16) Be aware of maintaining aseptic technique at all times throughout the procedure. If asepsis is accidentally broken, tell the surgeon and reglove.

(17) Remember to breathe! Many surgical assistants feel faint even having worked in the theatre for years. This is probably due to the fact that the assistant often has to stand very still in one position for long periods, concentrating hard whilst holding a particular body part. Adjusting body weight from one foot to the other is also important to keep the circulation moving.

A good assistant is invaluable and will help speed up the surgery and therefore reduce anaesthetic time.

THEATRE PRACTICE

CHAPTER 16

STERILISING EQUIPMENT FOR THEATRE

Sterilisation is the destruction of all micro-organisms and spores. Surgical instruments and some of the equipment used during surgery must be sterile before use. There are various methods that can be employed to ensure effective destruction of pathogenic micro-organisms and their spores and it is the responsibility of the VN to be familiar with the various techniques and their suitability for different surgical equipment.

The method by which items may be sterilised will depend on:

- The material, e.g. plastic, fabric, metal
- The quantity and size of items
- Financial constraints and sterilising equipment available

Sterilising methods may be divided into five main categories:

Dry heat:	hot air oven
Moist heat:	autoclave
Gaseous:	ethylene oxide
Chemical:	gluteraldehyde
Irradiation:	gamma radiation

Table 16.1 shows different methods of sterilisation.

DRY HEAT

Very high temperatures kill micro-organisms and their spores by destroying cell protoplasm. This method of sterilisation has limited use mainly because of the high temperatures that are required causing damage to many materials. It is however, the method of choice for *waxes* and *oils*, which can not be sterilised using moist heat.

The items are placed (unpacked) on to metal trays within the oven and left for a minimum of 60 minutes at 180°C. The oven is heated by an electrical element and should preferably be fan-assisted to prevent cold spots within the oven leaving

Table 16.1　Different methods of sterilisation.

Item	Steam autoclave	Dry heat hot air oven	Chemical gluteraldehyde	Gas ethylene oxide	Radiation prepacked
Drapes	✓ with drying cycle			✓	✓
Swabs	✓with drying cycle			✓	✓
Gowns	✓with drying cycle			✓	✓
Gloves	✓with drying cycle			✓	✓
Surgical instruments	✓with drying cycle	✓	✓	✓	
Suture material	✓ nonabsorbable			✓	✓
Suture needles	✓	✓	✓	✓	✓
Rubber drainage tubes	✓may perish			✓	✓
Endotracheal tubes	✓ may perish		✓	✓	
Anaesthetic tubing and bags			✓	✓	
Aqueous fluids	✓				✓
Oils		✓			✓
Ointments		✓			✓
Scalpel blades	✓	✓	✓	✓	✓
Endoscopes			✓	✓	
Thermometer			✓	✓	
Clipper blades		✓	✓	✓	
Electrosurgical probes	✓	✓	✓	✓	
Cryosurgical probes		✓	✓	✓	
Orthopaedic internal implants	✓			✓	

some items unsterilised. Table 16.2 gives times and temperatures for sterilising items.

MOIST HEAT

Micro-organisms are destroyed by wet or dry heat. Bacterial spores show a greater resistance to dry heat than to moist heat.

Table 16.2   Hot air oven time and temperatures.

Item	Temperature	Time
Glassware and metal instruments	180°C	60 minutes
Powders and oils	160°C	120 minutes

The presence of moisture coagulates the critical cellular proteins and destroys them at lower temperatures.

When water boils at 100°C it turns into steam. By raising the pressure within a chamber, the temperature of steam is raised. The higher the pressure, the higher the temperature and so the length of time required to sterilise is reduced.

A steam jacket surrounds the central sterilising chamber of an autoclave. During the sterilising process, the pressure in the jacket is raised before steam is introduced into the main chamber. Pre-existing air in the chamber is pushed downward by the steam and expelled from the system through vents to the outside. When all the air is removed and the desired pressure reached, the heat produced by the steam penetrates the innermost layers of the equipment packs. Table 16.3 shows different possibilities for using an autoclave.

GASEOUS

Ethylene oxide liquid is contained in a glass ampoule which when opened releases a gas that kills micro-organisms by a process called alkylation (essential cellular metabolic reactions are blocked). It is particularly useful for equipment that is damaged by moist or dry heat. Items are individually packaged and placed into a polythene liner bag that is placed into the special 'Anprolene' chamber. The glass ampoule is positioned in the middle of the bag and the top is broken off to release the gas. The door of the chamber is then closed and locked for the required period of time (12 hours sterilisation time plus 2 hour purge cycle).

Table 16.3   Autoclave temperature, time and pressure combinations.

Temperature	Time	Pressure
121°C	15 minutes	103 kPa (15 psi)
126°C	10 minutes	138 kPa (20 psi)
134°C	3½ minutes	207 kPa (30 psi)

Strict safety regulations control the use of 'Anprolene', the manufacturer's safety recommendations and COSHH regulations must be observed.

CHEMICAL

Gluteraldehyde liquid is capable of destroying micro-organisms and their spores. Items are placed into a container filled with a gluteraldehyde solution and submerged for up to 24 hours, depending on the manufacturer's recommendations. It is essential to rinse the equipment thoroughly afterwards with sterile saline because of the toxic and irritant effect of gluteraldehyde. Gloves, face masks and protective eyewear should be worn whilst handling.

This method is suitable for materials that will tolerate little or no heat, e.g. certain plastic tubes and fibre optic equipment.

IRRADIATION METHOD

Beta and gamma rays may be used to sterilise most materials with the exception of certain plastic and rubber combinations. The equipment required to generate the radioactive rays is very expensive and there are strict safety controls that restrict its use exclusively to industry. Many of the prepacked surgical materials such as suture materials and gloves are sterilised by this method.

STERILISING INDICATOR SYSTEMS

Successful sterilisation will depend on various factors such as the correct preparation of the packs, correct loading and operation of the steriliser and adequate times for sterilisation. It is important to use an indicator every load to ensure that sterilisation of the equipment has actually occurred. Available methods are shown in Table 16.4.

PREPARATION OF EQUIPMENT FOR STERILISATION

All equipment and instruments should be cleaned, dried and lubricated as necessary prior to packaging in the most appropriate wrapping material.

THEATRE PRACTICE

Table 16.4 Sterilising indicator systems.

Indicator	Action
Bowie-Dick tape	Impregnated with chemical stripes that change to dark brown when an adequate temperature has been reached (121°C). The tape responds only to temperature changes, irrespective of times and pressures.
Browne's tubes	Browne's tubes are small glass tubes partially filled with a liquid that changes colour from orange to green in response to the correct temperature being maintained for a required length of time. Browne's tubes are available for use in both autoclaves and hot air ovens and different tubes respond to the various ranges of temperatures 121, 126 134 and 180°C.
TST indicator strips	Strips of card with an indicator spot that changes colour (yellow to dark blue) in response to time, temperature and pressure. Must use the correct strip for a particular time/pressure/temperature setting.
Indicator spots	Plastic/paper pouches are available for packing items for sterilisation. Each bag is printed with two indicator spots, one is sensitive to ethylene oxide and the other is sensitive to moist heat.
Spore tests	Impregnated with dried bacterial spores. Following the autoclave cycle, the spore tests are sent for culture. If sterilisation has been effective, there will be no growth of any micro-organisms. Results from this test are not immediate.

The ideal wrapping material should be permeable to steam or gas but not to microbes and it should be flexible and resistant to damage. Different types of wrapping material are shown in Table 16.5.

METHOD OF PACKAGING

Always place instruments in the packaging, so that when the package is opened, the handles are facing out first. This enables the surgeon to take the instrument by the handles. Place instrument into autoclave bag so that the handles are facing the opening tabs.

Instruments and packed equipment should not be 'dropped' onto the instrument trolley but should be opened and passed to the surgeon or scrubbed assistant.

Always cover sharp tips or ends of equipment with a protective cover. (Special autoclave rubber tips are available or wrap a gauze swab over the end. Plastic syringe cases can be autoclaved and they make useful containers for needles, etc.)

LABELLING OF PACKS

All packages must be labelled with:

Table 16.5 Types of wrapping materials.

Material	Uses
Nylon film	Nylon film is designed particularly for use in autoclaves, it comes on a roll, in a variety of widths that can be cut to the desired length. It is relatively cheap and reusable although it starts to become brittle after several reuses. It is transparent which allows easy identification of the instruments inside and is waterproof.
Peelable pouches (Seal and Peel)	These are disposable pouches which are naturally more expensive than film. However, they have many benefits, including: • They are easy to open • Come in a variety of sizes • Are transparent (on one side) • Can be used with autoclave or ethylene oxide • Have sterilising indicator spots on the packet
Paper	Large sheets or rolls of a slightly elastic, crepe paper is available for wrapping around kits of instruments. It is water-resistant and can be cut to the required size.
Textiles	Certain cotton textiles (such as drapes and towels) can be used to wrap instrument packs. The advantage being that they are reusable and conforming. However, cotton is not water-resistant and it is better to use with paper outer covering.
Metal drums	Metal drums of various sizes are available and equipment may be placed directly inside these and sterilised. They are expensive to buy initially, however they can be reused forever. Their main disadvantages are that they are too large for most practice table-top sterilisers and they are often multi-used, therefore the rest of the kit is contaminated when opened.
Boxes and cartons	Corrugated plastic boxes with lids and a range of sizes are available for use in autoclaves. They are water resistant, reusable for many years and are particularly useful for complete kits and those containing specialised collections of equipment (e.g. orthopaedic kits).

- Date
- Name of piece of equipment or name of kit
- Name or initials of the person who packed the equipment

STORAGE OF PACKS

The way equipment is packed and stored will affect the shelf life of packs. A separate area should be available for storage of sterilised equipment, which is dust-free and away from contaminated articles. As a general rule, packed instruments may be considered sterile for up to six weeks, after which time they should be resterilised. Extremes of temperature, humidity and excessive handling will shorten the shelf life of the packs.

The most recently sterilised items should be placed behind older packs so that the older packs can be used first.

METHOD OF FOLDING SURGICAL GOWN FOR STERILISATION

(1) Lay the gown on a flat surface, with the outside of the gown facing upwards
(2) Smooth the front ties and place down the gown
(3) Fold the sleeves into the centre of the gown
(4) Fold one back flap into the centre of the gown
(5) Fold the second back flap into the centre of the gown
(6) Smooth down the back flap ties
(7) Fold into an accordion pleat
(8) Place folded gown into sterilising package

CHAPTER 17

CARE OF SURGICAL INSTRUMENTS

SURGICAL INSTRUMENTS

Most surgical instruments in veterinary practice are made of stainless steel. The different metals used make them resistant to corrosion and with correct usage, careful handling and thorough maintenance, instruments can last for many years.

Instruments have three different finishes, a mirror finish, which has been highly polished and makes the instrument very resistant to corrosion, a satin finish, which is designed to avoid the glare of the mirror finish instruments, and ebony finish, which eliminates glare completely. Tungsten carbide may be inserted into the tips and jaws of some instruments to provide an extremely hard-wearing surface, which can be replaced. These instruments usually have gold handles. Blue instruments, made of titanium, are used for some fine ophthalmic instruments because they are very light and hard wearing.

Colour coding instruments with special autoclavable tape will ensure that instruments are packed into their appropriate kits and reference cards listing specific instruments for each surgical procedure will make sure that all instruments are gathered up prior to surgery.

The role of the VN is extremely important in the care and maintenance of instruments and theatre equipment. If cared for, maintained properly and used only for their intended purposes they can last for up to 10 years.

Most instruments are made of stainless steel, which is an alloy of several metals; iron, carbon and chromium. The chromium element is what makes the steel resistant to corrosion.

In their manufacture, instruments go through various processes to increase their durability:

- The degree of hardness is achieved by subjecting the alloy to various degrees of heat

THEATRE PRACTICE

- They are placed into nitric acid which clears the metal of foreign matter or debris and also helps to form a protective corrosive-resistant chromium oxide layer

CARE AND MAINTENANCE OF INSTRUMENTS

- Instruments must only be used for the purpose for which they were intended
- Handle instruments carefully, never throw or drop them
- All new instruments must be cleaned, lubricated and sterilised before use
- Check hinged instruments for movability, all box joints should work smoothly
- Send blunt cutting instruments and drill bits away for re-sharpening
- Place protective tips over sharp and delicate instruments when not in use

PROCEDURE FOR CLEANING INSTRUMENTS

(1) *Never* leave instruments dirty for long periods of time. (The blood causes corrosion and staining of the instruments.)

(2) Place instruments in cold or lukewarm water with a mild detergent (e.g. washing up liquid) or preferably into a special surgical cleaning solution such as *Medigene*™, as soon as possible.

(3) *Never* leave the instruments to soak for long periods of time. Tap water may leave deposits on the instruments and sterile saline corrodes stainless steel. Ideally use distilled and deionised water or surgical cleaning solution.

(4) Wearing gloves, use a soft bristle brush to remove gross debris, pay particular attention to the ratchet mechanism, and the jaws of forceps.

(5) An ultrasonic cleaner may then be used if available (up to 90% of debris is removed after a 5 minute cycle).

(6) Always place the instruments with their joints open into the cleaner.

(7) Rinse instruments in cold water to remove detergent agent.

(8) Dry the instruments as much as possible, paying attention to joints and ratchet mechanisms. Place in warm area if possible to help dry (on top of boiler or heated cabinet if available).
(9) Lubricate instruments especially joints and ratchets with instrument milk or spray. (If instrument milk is used, the instruments do not need to be dried first.)
(10) Check the instruments thoroughly before sterilising (for any damage to joints, blades, ratchet mechanisms).
(11) Instruments should not be marked by etching methods as this will destroy the protective chromium layer.

COMMONLY USED INSTRUMENTS

Nurses should be able to recognise commonly used instruments and understand their use. A comprehensive list is given in Table 17.1.

FURTHER READING

Tracey, D.L. (1994) *Mosby's Fundamentals of Veterinary Technology, Small Animal Surgical Nursing*, 2nd edn. Mosby, USA.
Slatter, D. (1993) *Textbook of Small Animal Surgery*. WB Saunders & Co, London.

THEATRE PRACTICE

THEATRE PRACTICE

Table 17.1 Commonly used surgical instruments.

Instrument type	Example	Use
Scalpel handles	Bard-Parker	Holding scalpel blades
Needle holders	Mayo–Hegar Olson–Hegar Gillies McPhail Bruce-Clarke	Should be able to hold on to an appropriately sized needle without allowing rotation. Combination of holders and scissors (Gillies, Olson–Hegar)
Scissors	Metzenbaum Mayo – (straight or curved) Lister (bandage) Spencer (stitch) Potts	Use Mayo for dense tissue and Metzenbaum for more delicate dissecting Specialist types (Potts) angled for cardiovascular work. Classified by their blade points: sharp/blunt sharp/sharp blunt/blunt
Haemostats	Halstead Mosquito Kelly Crile Spencer-Wells	Range from fine mosquito to sturdier forceps often used for bone manipulation. Always check alignment and ratchet mechanism.
Tissue forceps	Allis Babcock Lane Doyen bowel clamp	Allis are fairly traumatic – do not use on skin or hollow organs. Babcocks – slightly less traumatic.
Thumb forceps	Semkin	Plain or with teeth to grip the tissue.
Dressing tissue	Adson Brown-Adson DeBakey Cooley Jeans	DeBakey and Cooley are atraumatic for cardiovascular work.
Towel clips	Backhaus Jones Cross action	Secures drape to skin (should be sharp). Do not remove once it has been placed as it breaks sterility.
Pin vise	Jacobs chuck	Holds Steinman pins and Kirschner wires
Bone saw	Gigli saw	
Retractors:	Hohmann	
Hand-held	Langenbeck	
Self-retaining	Malleable Gelpis Wests Travers Gosset	Allow adequate visualisation. Care must be taken not to trap intestines or nerves. Swabs may be used with abdominal retractors.

THEATRE PRACTICE

	Finochietto	
	Turvier	
	Balfour	
Bone-holding forceps	Lowman Spin(speed) lock Reduction	Used to manipulate and hold fragments of bone in place. With or without ratchets.
Rongeurs	Lempert Stille Luer Kerrison	Bone 'nibblers'. Must be used correctly or the jaws will blunt and become pitted. Kerrison rongeurs are used for fine spinal work.
Bone-cutting forceps	Liston Ruskin	Cutting bone
Periosteal elevators	Asif Freer	Used for reflecting the muscle from the bone.
Osteotomes	Lambotte	Both used for cutting into bone. Used with a mallet.
Chisels	Stille	
Curettes	Volkmann Sprat	Designed for scraping tissue from cavities or collecting cancellous bone grafts. Fine curettes are used for removing calcified disc material.
Trephines	Michel	Used for bone biopsies or for collecting cancellous bone grafts.
Ovariohysterectomy hook	Snook Covault	
Suction piece	Yankauer Frazier Ferguson Poole	For removing fluid or blood from the surgical field. Some come with an inner stylet to prevent blockage.

SECTION 3
SURGICAL NURSING

CHAPTER 18

ASSISTANCE DURING CAESAREAN SECTION (C-SECTION, HYSTEROTOMY)

Caesarean section is the delivery of fetuses via a laparotomy and further incision into the uterus. These patients are frequently seen late at night or in the early hours of the morning. This results in limited staff availability and tired workers. It is important that the VN is fully familiar with the procedure so that he or she can go into 'automatic mode'. This will help to prevent important aspects of care and treatment being overlooked or forgotten about. All of the equipment needed should be prepared beforehand because the VN will be too busy with the offspring to run around getting things later.

The VN must be fully competent in all of the activities surrounding a caesarean operation, including:

- Setting up and preparing appropriate surgical equipment
- Preparing appropriate anaesthetic equipment
- Preparing appropriate bedding and accommodation facilities for the dam and litter following surgery
- Preparing equipment and drugs for use during caesarean surgery
- Anaesthesia of the dam
- Receiving the neonate from the surgeon and managing the first essential steps of postparturient care
- Caring for neonates until dam recovers from anaesthesia
- Observation of the dam until full anaesthetic recovery

INSTRUMENTS

A general kit should provide all the instruments necessary for this procedure. Additional gauze swabs and large abdominal swabs should be prepared.

A box (e.g. a large, disinfected litter tray), hot water bottle or heat pad and plentiful supply of towels will be required for management of the offspring.

ANAESTHESIA

The aims of anaesthesia are to:

- Ensure adequate oxygenation (intubate)
- Maintain normovolaemia (intravenous fluids)
- Minimise depression of neonate during surgery and post-operatively (use short acting induction agent, e.g. propofol, and keep maintenance agent as low as possible, avoid using nitrous oxide)
- Minimise depression of the dam during surgery and post-operatively (require quick recovery)

Note: There is a potentially very dangerous situation with the mother immediately after the removal of the offspring from the uterus. The uterus, which previously occupied a large volume in the abdomen suddenly, greatly reduces in size causing a dramatic change in the dam's circulation. At this point, the animal is highly susceptible to shock and it is essential that her vital signs – heart rate, pulse quality, colour, etc. – are monitored. Intravenous fluids may be advisable throughout the procedure. A shock rate (20 ml/kg/hour) can be given immediately prior to, during and for a short time after the removal of the uterus and fetuses.

RECEIVING THE NEONATE FROM THE SURGEON

The surgeon will remove the puppy from the uterine horns and want to pass it on quickly so that he or she can continue on with the surgery.

The VN holds a towel in both hands and allows the surgeon to 'drop' the neonate into the open towel without contaminating the surgeon. The VN must then take the following steps quickly and efficiently:

(1) Using the roughness of the towel, break open the fetal membranes from around the neonate's head and body.
(2) Wipe the mouth and nose area with the towel to remove most of the fluid.
(3) Check to ensure a heart rate. (If present continue steps 4–12. If absent, follow resuscitation procedure.)
(4) Use a cotton bud to gently prize open the mouth and use it to wipe away the fluid inside the mouth – go in as far as pharynx area.

SURGICAL NURSING

(5) Use the towel to roughly rub the neonate to stimulate respiration.
(6) Respiration should now occur. Usually, a sharp, short inhalation is followed by short period of apnoea – keep rubbing neonate to stimulate (remember, they will still have the cardiorespiratory depressant effects of the anaesthetic agents).
(7) By now, the surgeon is probably ready to pass on another neonate so follow the above procedure.
(8) Place the first neonate into a box or large litter tray with hot water bottle/heated corn pad and clean bedding and keep checking it whilst sorting out the next neonate.
(9) Place new neonates next to the one before and at every opportunity, keep rubbing them to help stimulate them, help keep them warm and dry off their fur.
(10) Keep following the procedure shown above until all of the litter has been delivered.
(11) If there are more people around, e.g. the owner (!) get them to rub the neonates with a towel. By now they should be squeaking quite loudly.
(12) When all the neonates are delivered safely, tie off the umbilicus with gut suture material about 1 cm from the abdominal wall and cut just distal to the ligature.

ACTION IN THE EVENT OF APNOEA OR RESPIRATORY DEPRESSION

If there is a heartbeat but the neonate does not start breathing by stage 6, these next few steps should be taken:

(1) Hold neonate so that head is lower than the rest of the body to enable fluid to drain out. Reswab mouth using cotton bud or pipette
(2) Administer respiratory stimulant, e.g. doxopram hydrochloride (Dopram-V™). This is most frequently given orally by placing 1–2 drops under the tongue. Do not overdose.
(3) Gently blow down the nose and mouth (avoid direct contact) to provide oxygen
(4) Continue to stimulate the neonate by rubbing its entire body with the towel
(5) Continue to check for the presence of a heart beat
(6) Continue until regular respiratory efforts are maintained

ACTION TO TAKE IF THERE IS NO HEART BEAT

In some cases, the neonates have already died before the cae-sarean surgery and cardiovascular resuscitation is not indicat-ed. However, occasionally, there may not be a heart beat due to the depressant effects of the anaesthetic agents and cardiac massage can be performed:

(1) Place thumb and first finger on either side of the thorax over the position of the heart (if unsure, use point of elbow as a guide)

(2) Squeeze the thorax using firm, fast and regular move-ments (the neonates normal heart rate is over 200/min, so there is no way this rate can be achieved so aim to squeeze as quickly as possible in an effective way)

(3) Every 15 seconds or so, check for the presence of a heart beat and stimulate respiration as detailed above

(4) Check the neonate for obvious abnormalities that may be hindering attempts

(5) Continue until success or otherwise instructed to stop

PHYSICAL EXAMINATION OF THE NEONATE

When the entire litter has been delivered, a quick physical ex-amination can be performed to ensure the health of the young. It is essential to be aware of the huge differences in the values of the vital signs compared with adult animals of the same spe-cies. The normal values for the puppy and kitten in the first week of life are:

- Heart rate   220/min
- Respiration   15–40/min
- Temperature   34–36°C (94–97°F)

POSTSURGERY

A more detailed examination of the young should be per-formed to detect the presence of abnormalities including con-genital deformities.

Some dams will not accept the young after a caesarean. This may be overcome by waiting until she is recovered adequately from anaesthesia before placing them in the nest.

Avoid disturbing the dam but quietly and frequently observe the dam until she is sufficiently co-ordinated not to damage the young and all of the pups or kittens are suckling.

If possible, place the mother and offspring in a warm isolated area away from other noisy animals and human activity.

SURGICAL NURSING

CHAPTER 19

DENTISTRY

Periodontal disease affects more than 85% of dogs and cats over 3 years of age and although dentistry is a relatively new phenomenon to veterinary practice, many practices spend 25% or more of each day's operating time carrying out dental procedures.

This has opened up a new role for the VN who plays a part in both the education of the client regarding tooth care and oral hygiene, and also working with the patient and maintaining dental equipment. With the changes to the Veterinary Surgeons Act, VNs have more flexibility within dentistry and many practices have a specific *dental nurse*, who carries out mouth examinations and descaling.

It is therefore essential that the VN is fully familiar with the terminology, anatomy and physiology associated with the oral cavity and the nursing considerations of the patient undergoing dental treatment.

COMMON TERMS AND CONDITIONS

PERIODONTAL DISEASE

An inflammatory response caused by residual food, bacteria and calcium deposits (tartar) that collect in the spaces between the gum and lower part of the tooth crown. If left untreated, infection can spread to the bone in which the teeth are rooted. The bone then resorbs and the teeth are slowly detached from their supporting tissues.

HALITOSIS

Bad breath, which can be due to dental disease or uraemia.

DENTAL CALCULUS (TARTAR)

A combination of calcium phosphate and carbonate with organic matter, deposits in a hard covering on to the tooth surface

GINGIVITIS

Inflammation of the gums. There are numerous causes but it can lead to periodontitis.

CARIES

Erosion of tooth enamel because of bacteria from trapped food. Oxytetracyline given to pregnant bitches will affect the puppies' enamel causing pitting and yellowing of teeth and distemper also causes pitting and discoloration of the enamel in young dogs.

FRACTURED TEETH

This can be caused by stone chewing. The teeth may need removing or repairing if painful.

MALAR (CHEEKBONE) ABSCESS

Infection of the tooth root of the upper carnassial tooth.

MALOCCLUSION

This refers to malposition of the teeth resulting in the faulty meeting of the teeth or jaws. Malocclusion of the incisors is a common defect in all species and inherited in many dog breeds such as the brachycephalic breeds. With malocclusions in dogs and cats, abnormal striking of the teeth results in abnormal enamel wear.

In mammals with open-rooted teeth (e.g. rodents) malocclusion is a problem because their incisors do not meet to cause the continual grinding down of their teeth that is required to prevent overgrowth and consequently dysphagia. In such cases, the incisors must be clipped or filed throughout life.

TREATMENT OF PERIODONTAL DISEASE

The following equipment should be prepared and set up prior to any dental procedure:

- Ultrasonic dental machine containing a 0.2% chlorhexidine wash/coolant solution
- Dental polisher
- Dental forceps, hand-held scalers and curettes
- Mouth gag of appropriate size for the animal
- Pharyngeal packs
- Small pieces of damp cotton wool for cleaning debris
- Dental polish
- Fluoride solution
- Towels and grids to allow drainage of excess fluid from the mouth

TOOTH EXTRACTION

This is an uncertain area of the Veterinary Surgeons Act and it will be very much up to each practice's policy whether they allow their qualified nurses to extract teeth. Veterinary nurses should bear in mind that there are many hazards associated with a problem extraction including gum damage, broken tooth roots and fractured jaws. Unless the tooth can be pulled out with the fingers, it is probably best left to the veterinary surgeon, who is after all the one who will decide which, if any, teeth need to be removed.

SCALING

The current standard treatment of periodontal disease is to scale the teeth to remove supragingival plaque and calculus that attaches to the root surface. If large deposits of calculus are present, the worst of it can be removed using dental forceps or rongeurs to snap off as much as possible. If this technique is carried out incorrectly, damage to the crown, enamel or gum tissue can occur.

Once the worst of it is removed, an ultrasonic or sonic tooth descaler can be used. These tools work by vibrating a scaling tip at a high frequency over the tooth surface. This provides a fast method of scale removal but a certain amount of heat is generated which can cause tooth damage by causing pulp hyperthermia. When using these machines it is important to follow the guide below:

Sonic/ultrasonic tooth scaling

- Never spend more than 5–10 seconds per tooth. If necessary, go onto the next tooth and return to the original tooth in 10 seconds
- Never press hard with the tip of the scaler
- Never push the tip under the gumline (unless it is specially designed to do so)
- Hold the probe in a pen like grip and apply the tip side-on to the tooth (see manufacturer's instructions)

The desired affect is to achieve no visible debris on the tooth and the tooth surface is felt to be smooth and devoid of deposits and overhangs.

Hand scalers may be used instead of or in conjunction with powered equipment if desired. When properly performed, some dentists say that hand scaling is preferable to ultrasonic scaling because it causes less damage to the tooth structure. However, special training on hand scaling is required. They are held using a pen grip and should be sharpened after each use. They should never be used under the gum line.

After scaling has been completed on all aspects of the tooth surface, use a periodontal probe to feel for subgingival calculus and pockets greater than 3–5 mm in depth. Note pocket depths on the dental record.

Any remaining tartar from the root surface should be removed using subgingival curettes. If left, remaining tartar leaves an inflammatory focus and the disease will continue to deepen the periodontal pockets.

These half-moon shaped tips should be pushed into the bottom of the pocket and pulled upwards to remove the subgingival tartar. Overlapping strokes round the tooth in one direction and then again in the other should be performed to remove all of the calculus.

POLISHING

Polishing is an essential part of the cleaning and scaling process because it smoothes out the tiny pits and fissures on the tooth enamel which are created by the scaling process.

Most dental machines have a separate hand piece to which a disposable rubber cup is attached. A prophy paste is used in combination with a short (no more than 5–7 seconds on each tooth) light polishing of each tooth. The rubber cups should be allowed to flare out on the tooth surface so that both the supragingival and subgingival crown enamel is polished. The cup should be thrown away after each patient.

RINSING

After polishing, rinse any remnants of prophy paste and other debris (e.g. calculus) from the mouth and subgingival area. A 0.2% solution of chlorhexidine in a syringe with a blunted 21 g needle should be used to flush the gingival pockets around each tooth.

FLUORIDE TREATMENT

It has been recommended that a final application of fluoride (FluroFoam™ mousse) should be sprayed into the mouth and left for 2 minutes before being washed off. This helps to harden the enamel and desensitise the exposed dentine.

DENTAL CHART

A dental chart should be used to make notes about the amount of dental plaque, gingivitis and calculus together with information about pocket depth, missing teeth, extracted teeth, malocclusions and gingival recession.

These charts are available from most suppliers of veterinary dental equipment. They show a lateral and occlusal view of the mouth and each quarter of the mouth is given a number from 1 to 4. (1 = right upper, 2 = left upper, 3 = left lower and 4 = right lower). The numbering of the teeth starts from the midline, with the central incisor as 1.

ANAESTHETIC CONSIDERATIONS

Always ensure that a cuffed endotracheal tube is used and the cuff is inflated. Pack the pharynx with swabs (special foam sponges with string attachments are available, *Metropacks™*).

The head should be kept lower during the procedure if possible to allow all fluids to drain out of the mouth

The head must be kept lower during the recovery period, until full consciousness is regained. Remember to remove pharyngeal pack at the end of the procedure

PERSONAL HYGIENE AND SAFETY

Wear protective mask, disposable gloves and safety goggles during dental procedures to protect you from contact with the aerosol droplets created by the ultrasonic cleaner, which contain high numbers of bacteria.

EQUIPMENT MAINTENANCE

Hand instruments should be carefully washed in a proprietary instrument cleaner immediately after use and then dried thoroughly. Scalers and subgingival curettes should be sharpened with an Arkansas stone and oil before being autoclaved and stored in a perforated metal dental instrument tray.

The powered equipment requires cleaning after use. The unit, cables and hand pieces should be wiped down with a cleaning fluid and disinfectant. A couple of drops of the manufacturer's oil or lubrication should be placed into the inlet port of the hand piece. Remove the turbine from the high-speed hand piece and spray with an aerosol lubricant into the opening of the turbine. Replace and apply pressure to the footpad to ensure the oil penetrates the workings of the machine.

Release the pressure from the water tank and empty and allow to dry thoroughly.

SURGICAL NURSING

CHAPTER 20

SKIN SUTURING TECHNIQUES

CHARACTERISTICS OF SUTURE MATERIAL

- Knot security: how many 'throws' are required
- Capillary action: its ability to suck up fluid along its length
- Tissue drag: friction that occurs when throwing a knot
- Memory: ability to retain shape
- Chatter: friction caused when it passes over itself
- Sterilisation: how it can be sterilised
- Tissue reaction: irritant effect on tissues
- Elongation: stretchiness before breaking
- Tensile strength: strength before it breaks

CLASSIFICATION OF SUTURE MATERIALS

In the past many different materials were used to make sutures including intestinal tissue and kangaroo tendons, however, these days the most commonly used materials are synthetic although there are still a few natural products in use such as gut and silk.

A suture is classified in three ways depending on what it is made of:

- Absorbable or nonabsorbable
- Natural or synthetic material
- Monofilament or multifilament

ABSORBABLE SUTURES

- Lose their tensile strength between 10 and 40 days
- Are totally absorbed between 40 and 180 days
- Are absorbed by either phagocytosis or hydrolysis

- Natural absorbable sutures are removed by phagocytosis and produce some tissue reaction
- Synthetic absorbable sutures are removed by hydrolysis (broken down by fluid) and so there is minimal tissue reaction
- Are used for wound closures where long-term support is not needed

Examples:

- Plain and chromic surgical gut
- Polyglycolic acid: Dexon
- Polyglactin: Vicryl and Vicryl *Rapide*
- Polydioxanone: PDS II
- Polyglyconate: Maxon

NONABSORBABLE SUTURES

- Maintain their tensile strength > 60 days
- Become encapsulated in tissue
- Can be used where prolonged mechanical support is required, e.g. skin closure and slow-healing tissues

Examples:

- Linen
- Silk: Mersilk
- Polyamide: Ethilon and Supramid
- Polypropylene: Prolene
- Stainless steel: Dermalene

COMMON SUTURE MATERIALS

ABSORBABLE

Surgical gut
'Catgut' is made from the submucosa of small intestine of sheep and the intestinal serosa of cattle. There are two types: *plain gut*, which has no coating, and *chromic gut*, which has been tanned with chromic salts to slow the rate of absorption and reduce tissue reaction.

- Absorbable
- Natural

- Monofilament/multifilament
- Absorbed by enzymatic degradation and phagocytosis.
- Causes very little tissue reaction
- Absorbs fluids and swells
- Tensile strength 7–10 days (plain) and 17–21 days (chromic)

Polyglycolic acid – *Dexon*

- Absorbable
- Synthetic
- Multifilament
- Inert polyester
- Absorbed by hydrolysis
- Loses 80% strength by 14 days
- Absorbed in 40–60 days
- Braided (Dexon-S is coated)
- Some chatter
- A lot of tissue drag
- Poor knot security
- Very little tissue reaction

Polyglactin – Vicryl

- Absorbable
- Synthetic
- Multifilament
- Absorbed by hydrolysis
- Loses 50% strength by 14 days
- Maintains wound support 28–35 days (14 days for *Rapide)*
- Absorbed by 60–90 days (42 days for *Rapide)*
- Braided and coated
- Some tissue drag
- Very little tissue reaction
- Moderate knot security

Polydioxanone – PDS II

- Absorbable
- Synthetic
- Monofilament
- Absorbed by hydrolysis
- Retains 50% strength by 28 days

- Totally absorbed at 180 days
- Monofilament therefore less tissue drag
- Very little tissue reaction
- Very 'springy' with high memory
- Good knot security as it 'deforms' when tied

NONABSORBABLE

Silk – Mersilk

- Nonabsorbable
- Natural
- Multifilament
- Braided or twisted
- May be coated to minimise capillarity
- Loses 30% strength by 14 days
- Loses 60% strength by 30 days
- Excellent handling properties, knot security
- Main disadvantage is tissue reaction

Polypropylene – Prolene

- Nonabsorbable
- Synthetic
- Monofilament
- High tensile strength, but may stretch and fracture
- Poor handling qualities
- Reduced knot security
- High memory
- Virtually no tissue reaction
- Little tissue drag

Polyamide (nylon) – Ethilon and Supramid

- Nonabsorbable
- Synthetic
- Monofilament/multifilament
- High tensile strength
- Very little tissue reaction
- Impregnated with wax to reduce capillarity
- Average knot security
- Very little tissue drag

METALS – STAINLESS STEEL OR TANTALUM

- Nonabsorbable
- Monofilament or multifilament
- Difficult to handle
- High tensile strength
- Kinks easily
- No tissue reaction
- No tissue drag
- Difficult to knot
- Very good knot security

ALTERNATIVES TO SUTURE MATERIALS

STAPLES

May be used for skin wound closure, for lung lobectomies, liver biopsies and bowel resection. They are expensive and need special equipment for the application of the staples. The main benefit is that they are extremely quick and provide good closure when used in internal organs.

ADHESIVE TAPES

Are available for wound closure but they are expensive and do not stick well to moist skin or skin with animal hair stubble.

TISSUE GLUE

Cyanoacrylate monomers are used to glue skin edges together, but they are toxic and have been shown to cause a granuloma reaction.

SELECTION OF SUTURE MATERIALS

EXAMPLES OF APPROPRIATE MATERIALS FOR PARTICULAR BODY TISSUES

- Skin: Monofilament nylon, polypropylene
- Subcutis: Fine, synthetic, absorbable, e.g. Vicryl
- Fascia: Synthetic, nonabsorbable or PDS, Vicryl

- Muscle: Synthetic absorbable or nonabsorbable nylon or polypropylene for cardiac muscle
- Hollow viscus: Synthetic absorbable or polypropylene
- Tendon: Stainless steel, nylon, polypropylene
- Blood vessels: Polypropylene
- Nerves: Nylon or polypropylene

TISSUE HEALING RATES

When selecting an appropriate suture material for use in a particular body area, it is useful to consider the tissue healing rates of that area so that the most appropriate suture material can be selected:

- Skin: 7–10 days
- Fat: 5 days
- Muscle: 14 days
- Fascia: 42 days
- Serosa/mucosa: 2–3 days

SELECTION OF SIZE OF SUTURE MATERIAL

When selecting the size of the suture material, the VN should always aim to use the smallest diameter possible for each particular body part and the size of the animal.

The size of suture material is expressed using two different methods:

- Metric
- USP (US pharmacopoeia)

The metric figure refers to the diameter of the suture material in 0.1 mm.
For example:

- Actual size = 0.4 mm
- Metric size = 4
  - (Multiply actual size by 10)

USP	Metric
5–0	1
4–0	1.5
3–0	2
2–0	3
0	3.5
1	4
2	5
3	6

SUTURE NEEDLES

Made from stainless steel, occasionally coated with silicone to facilitate passage through the tissues.

The method of attaching the suture material to the needle may be either:

- Through an 'eye'
- Swaged

EYED NEEDLES

- Are reusable
- Can be used with any type or size suture material
- Are cheaper
- However, repeated sterilisation dulls cutting edges
- More bulky to go through tissues

Single-eye needles should never be double-threaded as the bulk of the suture material causes severe tissue drag.

SWAGED

- Suture material is attached directly
- Atraumatic to tissues
- Expensive
- Sharper
- Ensured sterility

SHAPE OF NEEDLES

Suture needles come in a variety of shapes:

- Straight (used for hand suturing – not to be used with needle holders)
- Half-curved
- Curved

The choice of needle shape is usually governed by the accessibility of the tissue to be sutured, and normally the more confined the operative site the greater the curvature required.

POINTS

Cutting needles can be used in very dense or tough tissues. They are designed to be used in the skin. They incise a hole larger than the needle shank, therefore reducing tissue drag.

Tapercut needles have a cutting tip on the point and a round body. They do not cut but spread the tissue and cause very little tissue trauma. They can be used in any type of tissue.

Roundbodied do not cut – they are designed to separate tissue fibres rather than cut them. They are used for nonfibrous tissue, soft tissue organs and any delicate tissue where the tissue fibres are split easily.

Reverse cutting needles look similar to cutting needles, but the difference is that the apex cutting edge is on the outside of the needle curvature. This improves the strength of the needle and increases its resistance to bending.

Spatulated needles are extremely fine with very sharp cutting edges. They are used primarily for ophthalmic work.

NEEDLE SIZE AND STRENGTH

Needle sizes come in a range:

- 4, 5, 6 … 22, 23, 24
- Coarse … fine

The diameter of the needle is a major factor in determining its strength, although the cross-sectional shape and type of wire are also important. The size of needle should be selected taking into consideration the tissue to be sutured, the size of the suture material required and the force required to push the suture needle through the tissue.

Most needles are designed so that they bend rather than break when they are over-stressed. This bending indicates that the needle has been used in a situation where a force has been applied which is greater than that for which it was designed. If bending occurs, the needle should be discarded rather than any attempt made to straighten it.

USE OF NEEDLE HOLDERS

The needle holder should be carefully selected to match the size of the needle being used. An overly large needle holder can cause damage and bend the needle.

The needle size and curvature should match the size of the tissue bite required. Use of too small a needle for a given tissue will lead to bending of the needle.

The needle holder should be in good condition – worn jaws result in needle rotation and instability of the needle.

The needle should be held only on the flattened area and should not be grasped near the needle point or attachment or eye area. Nonflattened needles should be grasped at approximately one third of the total needle length from the suture material end.

The force required to pass the needle through the tissues should be applied in the direction of the curvature of the needle.

The needle should be inserted into each side of the tissue separately and should not be used to bridge a wound.

SUTURE PATTERNS

The suture pattern used in any area depends on the wound tension and personal preference and expertise.

Suture patterns can be divided into:

• Interrupted
• Continuous sutures

They are further classified into:

• Simple
• Mattress
• Tension sutures

The most commonly used patterns are:

Simple interrupted

Used in many areas of the body they are easy to insert and maintain good tissue apposition. Occasionally, the wound edges may invert or if the sutures are placed too far apart, the wound will gape in between the sutures. See Fig. 20.1.

Simple continuous

This is often used to close subcutaneous tissues and skin. It is extremely quick to apply and gives good skin apposition. The major disadvantage with this technique is that a break in the suture line or knot will lead to total relaxation of the suture line and wound breakdown. See Fig. 20.2.

Horizontal mattress

This is used for skin closure, especially when the edges of the wound are under a certain amount of tension. See Fig. 20.3.

Vertical mattress

This is used as above. See Fig. 20.4.

Cruciate mattress

This is used for skin closure and provides good apposition of the wound edges. It is useful when there is moderate tension

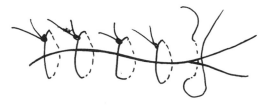

Fig. 20.1   Simple interrupted suture.

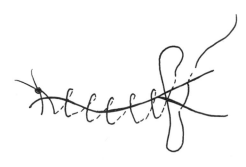

Fig. 20.2   Simple continuous suture.

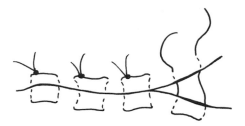

Fig. 20.3   Horizontal mattress suture.

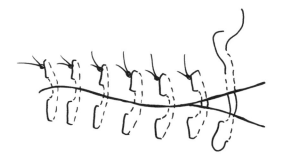

Fig. 20.4   Vertical mattress suture.

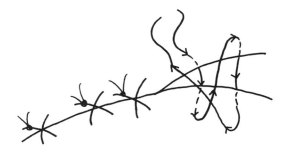

Fig. 20.5   Cruciate mattress suture.

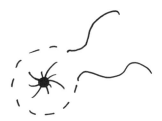

Fig. 20.6   Purse string suture.

and is quicker than using simple interrupted sutures. Removal is quicker as well. See Fig. 20.5.

Purse string suture

This is used to temporarily close an orifice (e.g. anus during surgery around that area) It is quick to apply and remove. See Fig. 20.6.

CHAPTER 21

PRACTICAL CARE OF WOUNDS

There are four main factors to consider in the management of wounds:

- The type of wound (classification)
- Initial treatment and care of wounds when first seen
- Continued management of wound with appropriate dressing materials
- Signs of wound breakdown and delayed healing

THE CLASSIFICATION OF WOUNDS

CLEAN

A surgical wound made under aseptic conditions. There is no break into a contaminated area such as the respiratory or gastrointestinal tract.

CLEAN-CONTAMINATED

Another surgical wound, made under aseptic theatre conditions, but where it incorporates an incision into a contaminated area such as the respiratory, gastrointestinal or urogenital tract. However, there has been no spillage of the contents of the contaminated area into the wound.

CONTAMINATED

As above but spillage has occurred from one of these contaminated areas into the wound. Also may occur in traumatic injury such as one immediately following a road traffic accident (RTA) or animal bite, where contaminants are present but not sepsis (yet).

DIRTY

An infected wound. Either from a surgical wound into an area
of the body containing bacteria such as the gut or from a contaminated traumatic wound over 6–8 hours old.

Note: Contaminated wounds can become dirty wounds if the
debris is not removed before 6–8 hours. This is called the 'golden
period'. This refers to the time it takes for bacteria to be implant-
ed somewhere and then begin to grow and multiply. This is why
it is so important to thoroughly flush and clean all wounds as
soon as possible, rather than leaving them until later.

THE INITIAL TREATMENT AND CARE OF WOUNDS WHEN FIRST SEEN AT THE CLINIC

Wound healing will not occur until debris and infections are
removed. Cleaning and decontamination of the wound is the
most effective way of reducing long-term bacterial contamination and should ideally be carried out in the first 6–8 hours
after injury.

Aggressive action should be taken to thoroughly lavage and
debride the wound. Ideally, this should be carried out in a
clean/sterile environment (e.g. theatre or theatre preparation
room).

WOUND CLEANING

(1) If the wound is older than 8 hours, obtain a swab for bacterial culture and sensitivity.

(2) Apply a water-soluble lubricating gel to the wound. This
makes it easier for the clipped fur to be removed from the
wound during lavage.

(3) Clip hair from around the wound. Use scissors for clipping the hair around the wound edges. (It may help to
wet the scissors with lubricating gel so that clipped hair
sticks to the scissors rather than falling in to the wound.)

(4) Lavage the entire wound with copious quantities of
warmed sterile, isotonic saline.

(5) If the wound is very contaminated, *warm* tap water may
be used initially to remove gross dirt, however, prolonged used of tap water will damage the exposed tissues
because of its osmolality.

(6)   Some people advocate the use of mild antiseptic solutions (2% povidone-iodine) but many antiseptic solutions are in fact an irritant to the tissues and their use has not been shown to be of any additional benefit to the long-term wound healing process.

(7)   Apply appropriate sterile dressing material and bandage.

Lavage technique

Use of a 20 or 30 ml syringe and 19 gauge hypodermic needle to lavage the wound has been shown to provide the ideal lavage pressure. High pressures run the risk of forcing debris and bacteria further into the wound and low pressures have been shown to provide ineffective lavage. Aerosol pumps, attached to drip bags, are commercially available and provide optimum lavage pressures.

Debridement technique

Debridement may be carried out on necrotic tissue using a sterile scalpel blade, scissors and forceps. This must be carried out in a sterile theatre environment. Layered, staged and en-bloc resection are methods of debridement and should only be carried out following training and instruction from the VS.

CONTINUED MANAGEMENT OF WOUNDS USING DRESSINGS AND BANDAGES

After the trauma of a wound, the fluid that is immediately released into the area dries out and forms a scab. A scab is the body's natural wound dressing, designed to protect the healing wound and prevent further contamination.

However, a scab will delay the healing process in two ways: it increases the amount of necrotic material within the wound and also means that the migrating epithelial cells have to force a route beneath the scab. Wounds that heal in this way are far more likely to scar.

The aim of wound management is to prevent the wound from drying out and prevent the formation of a scab. This allows the epithelial cells to migrate rapidly over the wound surface.

THE CONTACT LAYER (PRIMARY WOUND DRESSING)

There are many ways to classify wound-dressing materials. For example, the following terms are used:

- Dry dressings
- Moist dressings
- Wet dressings
- Impregnated gauze
- Adherent or nonadherent dressings

However, this is not really very important. What is important is that the VN knows what is available and what is most appropriate for a particular wound at each stage of its healing process.

DRY DRESSINGS (NONADHERENT)

Generally, dry dressings such as Melolin may be used on surgical wounds where the edges of the wound are held together. For most other types of wound, they have been shown to be detrimental to wound healing. They tend to adhere to the wound surface, causing pain and disruption of the healing processes upon removal.

DRY TO DRY

This method of dry to dry dressings has gone out of fashion. Their main application is for dirty, necrotic wounds that have lots of loose tissue and foreign matter to remove. Sterile surgical gauze is applied dry to the wound surface. When it is removed (each day), a layer of tissue is removed along with the necrotic material and debris.

The main reason for their discontinued use is that removal can be extremely uncomfortable if not painful for the patient and it is not just the necrotic tissue and debris that is removed. A certain amount of the healthy, healing cells are disrupted and removed. This type of dressing should never be used in wounds with good granulation and epithelialisation.

WET TO DRY

Wet to dry work in a very similar way to dry to dry dressings. The gauze swab is first soaked in sterile saline before being applied to the wound. This reduces the viscosity of wound exudate so that it may be absorbed more easily. The fluid then evaporates and the dressing becomes dry by the time it is removed, thus pulling away everything else with it.

These dressings have added disadvantages over dry to dry because the moist environment is conducive to bacterial growth and also the tissues surrounding the wound may become macerated if the dressing is too wet. The use of cold wetting solutions can cause discomfort to the animal.

IMPREGNATED GAUZE DRESSINGS

These are slightly less adherent than dry dressings but they do very little to actively promote wound healing. Examples include Jelonet, Grassolind.

POULTICE

A poultice is a paste or impregnated dressing that is applied to an area to draw out infection, they are used more widely in large animal medicine than in small animals. Animalintex is the most commonly used commercial poultice.

With such sophisticated materials available commercially, there is no need to continue using these outdated methods. Moist dressings are now the materials of choice.

MOIST DRESSINGS (NONADHERENT)

Moist wound dressings (hydrogels such as Intrasite and Biodress and hydrophilics such as Allevyn) are interactive dressing materials that are extremely useful in maintaining a moist wound environment. Their use has been shown to accelerate wound healing by providing an optimum wound temperature, encourage the migration of cells from the edges of the wound and encouraging cell mitosis. They are able to remove excess exudate and toxic components whilst giving protection from secondary infection. They are easy to remove and do not cause trauma or pain at dressing change.

Note: There is no single dressing material that can provide the optimum environment for all wounds or for the total healing stages of one wound, therefore it is important to select the most appropriate dressing for each wound at each particular stage of the healing process. This is why it's important for the

VN to research available products and keep up to date with new materials.

SIGNS OF WOUND BREAKDOWN AND DELAYED HEALING

It is absolutely essential that the VN is able to recognise the clinical signs of wound breakdown and delayed healing. The VN must be confident in examining wounds and reporting findings to the attending VS.

Clinical signs of wound breakdown include:

- Erythema
- Inflammation
- Discharge
- Separation of wound edges
- Interference of the wound by the patient
- System illness, e.g. pyrexia
- Change in wound colour (pale = reduced blood supply, dark/black = necrotic tissue)
- Malodour

Factors that affect the speed of wound healing include:

- The general physiological condition of the animal
- The nutritional status of the animal
- The blood supply to the wound area
- Presence of foreign material
- Presence of infection
- The site of the injury
- The tissue mobility

SECTION 4
ANAESTHESIA

CHAPTER 22

INTRODUCTION – EVALUATION OF THE PATIENT

Anaesthesia is a very important part of veterinary nurse training. Although it is the responsibility of the VS to choose appropriate drugs and to induce anaesthesia, monitoring the patient and ensuring the animal is kept asleep during the procedure is often the role of the VN. Therefore an understanding of the drugs used, the monitoring process and the equipment is very important.

PATIENT EVALUATION

A medical history should be obtained, with results from previous laboratory analysis and current body weight. All details must be recorded as a basis for comparison during and after surgery so that subsequent abnormalities can be detected quickly. All patients should be thoroughly evaluated prior to anaesthesia to assess not only the system affected by the primary disease but also the animal's general health. The VN must be confident in performing a general clinical examination. Many patients, particularly those undergoing routine, elective surgery, will be in good health and may be anaesthetised with minimal risks using standard anaesthetic protocols. Some patients, however, will be classified as medium to high-risk cases and will need to be stabilised and an anaesthetic regime designed appropriately. A note should be made of previous and current medication treatments (some medications may affect anaesthetic protocols or medication regimes). It may be useful in some cases to determine if the animal has had a blood transfusion in the past, as subsequent transfusion will require cross-matching.

Table 22.1 describes how to categorise an animal's physical status (from American Society of Anesthesiologists).

Table 22.1   Classes of risk from an animal's physical status.

Class	Animal condition
Class 1 – minimal risk	Normal healthy animals with no underlying disease, e.g. ovariohysterectomy, castration, hip dysplasia radiography
Class 2 – slight risk	Animals with mild systemic disturbances with no clinical signs of disease because they are able to compensate,e.g. neonate or geriatric animals, obese animals, animals with fractures but no shock, mild diabetes
Class 3 – moderate risk	Animals showing mild clinical signs associated with moderate systemic disease, e.g. anaemic, anorexic, moderately dehydrated patients, low-grade kidney disease, low-grade heart disease, and pyrexia
Class 4 – high risk	These are animals with pre-existing systemic disease or severe system disturbances, e.g. severe dehydration, shock, anaemia, uraemia, toxaemia, pyrexia, uncompensated heart disease
Class 5 – grave risk	Animals with a life-threatening system disease, e.g. moribund patients, advanced heart, kidney, liver, lung or endocrine disease, profound shock, severe trauma

LABORATORY TESTS

Animals undergoing elective surgery, class 1 and 2 patients, can usually be safely anaesthetised using routine techniques, however, laboratory screening tests (packed cell volume, total serum protein and blood urea nitrogen) may be useful to diagnose an animal with subclinical disease. Older animals, those undergoing long surgical procedures, trauma patients and animals with abnormal organ function will benefit from a general biochemical and haematological profile prior to surgery to minimise complications and to help choose an appropriate anaesthetic protocol.

Other tests and evaluation procedures such as radiography to assess lung function and electrocardiography to evaluate the heart may be indicated in the higher risk anaesthetic patients.

PATIENT STABILISATION

A certain number of cases requiring surgery will need some form of stabilisation prior to surgery, for example patients with hypovolaemic shock as a result of trauma (e.g. road traffic accident), septicaemia (e.g. pyometra) and endotoxaemia (e.g. gastric dilatation).

FLUID THERAPY

Fluid therapy is indicated in dehydration, trauma, shock or metabolic disease. By combining the information gained from an accurate history with evidence of any clinical signs associated with dehydration, the need for fluid therapy can be assessed.

Disturbances in the body's electrolytes and acid-base balance can produce a wide range of clinical signs. Large changes in pH may result in the animal becoming depressed and can be fatal. The aim of fluid therapy is to replace deficits and restore the electrolyte and acid-base imbalance that may have occurred. The fluid therapy protocol can be planned to take any changes into consideration, however, without the necessary analysing equipment an estimate may only be made using information gained from history, clinical examination and knowledge of disease processes.

FOOD AND WATER

It is usually recommended that food is withheld for 8–12 hours prior to induction of anaesthesia. Prolonged starvation is not appropriate in young animals or older animals with concurrent disease due to depleted liver glycogen reserves, which leaves the animal less able to withstand the stress of anaesthesia and surgery. Water, in the vast majority of cases, should only be withheld for 2 hours prior to anaesthesia and no longer to prevent the risk of dehydration and hypovolaemia.

PREMEDICATION

Pre-anaesthetic medication is frequently administered prior to induction of general anaesthesia for a number of reasons:

- To calm and control the patient
- To provide analgesia throughout surgery
- To reduce the amount of anaesthetic induction and maintenance agent required
- To produce a smooth induction of anaesthetic
- To reduce some of the unwanted side-effects of some of anaesthetic agents

ANAESTHESIA

- To ensure a smoother recovery from anaesthesia

A combination of sedatives/tranquillisers, analgesics and anticholinergic agents are most frequently used. There may well be a standard practice premedication protocol, which is suitable for most surgical cases. However, the choice of drugs will depend on the patient's physiological condition and the type of surgery to be performed.

The VN must be confident in calculating dose rates, be familiar with administration routes and be aware of common side-effects of the drugs used.

FACTORS DETERMINING CHOICE OF ANAESTHETIC DRUGS

(1) Facilities and drugs available
(2) Experience of the veterinary surgeon and nurse
(3) Postoperative facilities
(4) Species variation (Saffan can not be used in dogs, drug doses differ in different species)
(5) General condition of the animal and other diseases
(6) Age
(7) Temperament
(8) Breed peculiarities (Boxers and acepromazine)
(9) Proposed surgical procedure
    - Site
    - Need for muscle relaxation
    - Type (caesarean, thoracotomy)
    - Duration

INTRAVENOUS CATHETERISATION

If possible, an intravenous (I/V) catheter should be placed prior to surgery (this may be easier to carry out just before or at the time of premedication because of the hypotensive effect of acepromazine, which may make catheter placement more difficult). The presence of an I/V catheter line facilitates a smoother induction if an I/V agent is to be used and greatly reduces the risk of accidental perivascular injection. Intravenous fluid therapy can also be administered via this route. Should intravenous fluid therapy be deemed necessary during surgery, a preplaced catheter ensures quick and easy administration. Catheterisation also provides a swift route for drugs in the event of an anaesthetic emergency.

POSTOPERATIVE CARE

Postoperative care and observation of the patient is an essential part of the whole surgical procedure and should never be underestimated. The VN must be confident about which parameters to monitor and be aware of the common complications associated with each type of surgical procedure and each individual patient. Routinely, a temperature, pulse and respiration rate must be obtained and recorded every 15 minutes until a return to normal is seen. The patient should never be left unattended whilst the endotracheal tube is in place.

HYPOTHERMIA

Hypothermia is extremely common following anaesthesia and surgery due to the combined effects of the presurgical clip and scrub, cold anaesthetic gases administered via a nonrebreathing circuit, cold operating rooms and tables, a reduction in muscular activity during anaesthesia and an anaesthetic-induced decrease in the basal metabolic rate. It is also the most common cause of bradycardia following surgery. Reduction or preferably prevention of hypothermia is an important factor for a rapid recovery from anaesthesia and to prevent patient discomfort. Hypothermia slows down the metabolic rate and therefore the metabolism of anaesthetic drugs. External heat will be required in the hypothermic patient in the form of blankets, bubble wrap, heat pads and lamps but it must be remembered that the recumbent animal is unable to move away from any heat source and is at risk of burning. Direct contact with heat pads, hot water bottles and skin must be avoided.

During surgery, some simple techniques can be employed which will help to reduce hypothermia. These include:

- Warming all intravenous fluids
- Warming bags of saline used during open body cavity flushing
- Keeping surgery time to a minimum
- Maintaining a warm ambient operating room temperature (23°C)

- Using an in-circuit water vapour trapping device (Thermovent 600™, Portex Ltd) placed between the endotracheal tube and the anaesthetic circuit

Rapid increases in body temperature and hyperthermia should be avoided. Central nervous system damage can occur as a result of dehydration, hypotension and hypoxia. Frequent monitoring of peripheral and core temperature is therefore essential and once a return to normothermia is achieved, heat sources should be removed/turned off. As a guide, the patient may be warmed by at least 0.5°C per hour.

Measurement of a peripheral temperature is useful to provide information about the quality of peripheral perfusion. Under normal conditions in normal room temperature, peripheral temperature (measured between the third and fourth rear digits in the foot) is 2–5°C lower than core temperature. Temperature differences greater than this indicate vasoconstriction and poor peripheral perfusion associated with shock; the greater the difference, the more severe the changes.

POSTOPERATIVE PAIN

Observation of the patient's behaviour following surgery is important to detect signs of pain. It is well known that it is better to prevent pain than to treat it and that analgesic drugs are significantly more effective if administered before the onset of pain, (e.g. as part of the premedication and during anaesthesia). It is helpful to observe the animal's general behaviour before surgery so that the individual nature of each patient can be considered in postoperative pain assessment. Animals that are stressed and anxious will be more sensitive to pain. Gentle handling at all times during the patient's stay in the hospital and allowing the animal to recover in a quiet, dimly lit area will help to reduce stress.

At different stages in the recovery period, an animal may show different clinical signs of pain. In the initial stages there may be obvious signs such as howling, restlessness and thrashing around in the kennel. As the patient regains consciousness, clinical signs may become less obvious but may include some behavioural changes such as anorexia, failing to drink and groom and adopting an unusual posture.

Opioid analgesics provide the most effective means of pain control in small animals. Nonsteroidal anti-inflammatory drugs (NSAIDs) only relieve pain of low to moderate intensity. When used as analgesics, care must be taken when using NSAIDs especially in patients with renal, hepatic or cardiac dysfunction. Aspirin may decrease platelet aggregation and therefore cause increased bleeding times. It should not be used as preoperative analgesia.

ANAESTHESIA

CHAPTER 23

ENDOTRACHEAL INTUBATION

Endotracheal tubes provide a connecting link between the patients' airway and the anaesthetic system. It also maintains a patent airway and VNs must be confident in carrying out this procedure so that it may be performed efficiently in the event of an emergency.

TUBE SELECTION

- Sizes range from 2.5 mm to 16 mm in small animals and 16 mm to 40 mm in large animals
- The tube should extend from the nose to a point level with the spine of the scapula
- Tubes should be cut to the correct length before use or this will increase the dead space
- Uncuffed tubes should always be used in cats as the trachea can be damaged easily by over-inflated cuffs
- A cuff also decreases the bore diameter
- Reinforced tubes help prevent kinking when the neck is flexed

INTUBATION TECHNIQUE

ASSISTANT RESTRAINING THE ANIMAL

(1) Restrain animal in sternal or lateral recumbency (depending on operator's preference.
(2) Extend the animal's neck.
(3) Open the animal's mouth with one hand, usually left hand if the animal is in left lateral recumbency. Avoid putting fingers in the animal's mouth – place thumb on left gum and index and middle finger on the other gum.

or

(1) Pass a tape strip in the mouth, behind the canines to hold the upper jaw open – especially useful in brachycephalic dogs and reduces the risk of the animal accidentally biting the assistant. See Fig. 23.1.

OPERATOR

(1) Always ensure there is adequate anaesthetic depth to ensure muscle relaxation of the upper airway.
(2) Select an appropriate size of endotracheal tube. Using a tube that is too large may cause laryngeal or tracheal trauma. A tube that is too small will enable the animal to breathe room air around the tube or allow aspiration of oral secretions.
(3) Check the length of the tube before use – from the nostrils to the manubrium. Cut the tube down if necessary.

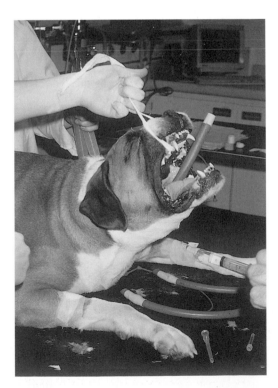

Fig. 23.1   Endotracheal intubation – holding the mouth open with bandage.

ANAESTHESIA

(4) Check the function of the cuff before intubating the animal.

(5) Lubricate the tracheal end of the tube with water or water soluble gel.

(6) Pull the animal's tongue forward out of the mouth with one hand, using one finger of the same hand to pull the mandible downwards to open the mouth as much as possible. Take care not to lacerate the ventral aspect of the tongue on the lower incisor teeth.

(7) If necessary position light source to view larynx. Place the tip of the laryngoscope blade at the base of the tongue and press the tip of the blade ventrally to expose the glottis.

(8) Apply local anaesthetic if necessary.

(9) Depress the epiglottis with the tip of the endotracheal tube.

(10) Hold the tube so that the bevel is in the vertical position in line with the vocal folds and cavity.

(11) Pass the end of the endotracheal tube through the glottis into the trachea.

(12) Once the bevel is positioned through the vocal folds into the larynx, turn the tube so that the curve of the tube matches the curve of the trachea.

(13) Continue to advance the tube so that its distal tip is level with the manubrium.

(14) The assistant places the animal's head gently onto the table.

(15) Check to ensure correct placement of tube (hold a small piece of W.O.W bandage in front of the tube and it should move during expiration).

(16) Tie and knot the prepared W.O.W tape strip to the endotracheal tube.

(17) Secure the tube in position by tying behind the ears or upper jaw depending on procedure to be performed or size of animal.

(18) Inflate the cuff if necessary, taking care not to over-inflate as this may reduce the internal diameter of the tube and cause tracheal damage. The bulb should inflate with gentle pressure, stop when more resistance is felt. Check by squeezing the reservoir bag on the circuit.

Notes:

• Generally, intubate cats with a noncuffed tube, a cuffed tube may cause damage to the cat's delicate trachea and will result in a smaller diameter tube having to be used.

- Do not over-inflate the tube as this may result in pressure necrosis of the tracheal epithelium or narrowing of the inner diameter.
- Forced intubation may cause damage to the larynx resulting in oedema, laryngeal spasm, vagal stimulation and cardiac arrhythmias.
- Local anaesthetic agent may be used in cats.

EXTUBATION

(1) Leave tube in place until the swallowing reflex returns.
(2) In the cat, the tube should be removed just prior to this to prevent laryngeal trauma.
(3) Ensure the cuff is deflated before removal.
(4) Pull the tongue forward and gently extend the neck.
(5) Observe patient to ensure airway remains clear.
(6) After use, the tubes should be washed and disinfected. Oral secretions should be removed from the inner lumen using a bottlebrush and the outside of the tube gently wiped. The whole tube should be rinsed with water and the cuff tested before leaving to soak for an appropriate time in disinfectant solution (e.g. Trigene).
(7) The tubes can be sterilised using ethylene oxide (Anprolene) and the latex tubes can be autoclaved although this quickly perishes the rubber.

CHAPTER 24

MONITORING GENERAL ANAESTHESIA

Monitoring general anaesthesia is a full-time responsibility and must not be combined with other duties or tasks. When an animal is anaesthetised, it is taken from a state of consciousness to unconsciousness, stopping at surgical anaesthesia before returning to consciousness again. When the VN monitors an animal during this time, he or she needs to be able to ensure that the animal remains stable at the surgical anaesthetic level. Overdose and failure to recognise signs of deepening of unconsciousness can lead to death. It is important to recognise the different signs associated with changing levels of unconsciousness in the patient, and be able to take the appropriate actions required. Early observation and appropriate intervention will help to ensure that minor problems do not turn into major anaesthetic emergencies. The patient should be checked frequently (at least every 5 minutes) and the results recorded on an anaesthetic chart. This record encourages regular checking of the patient, allows trends to be identified and provides evidence in the event of litigation. See Fig. 24.1 for detail of monitoring anaesthesia.

The patient should be watched particularly closely during induction and recovery from anaesthesia.

WHAT TO CHECK TO ASSESS 'DEPTH' OF ANAESTHESIA

- Respiratory system
- Cardiovascular system
- Reflexes
- Mucous membranes
- Temperature

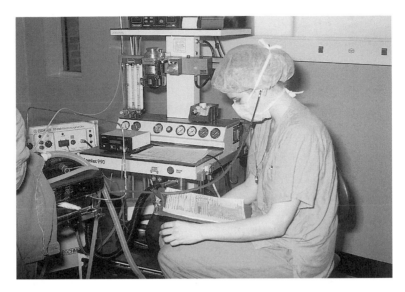

Fig. 24.1 Monitoring anaesthesia.

RESPIRATORY SYSTEM

It is important to ensure that there is a patent airway during anaesthesia, and that adequate ventilation is being achieved. The VN should check the respiration movements by looking at the bag on the anaesthetic machine. This enables the VN to monitor the respiratory rate without disrupting or touching the surgical drapes, etc. and more importantly, indicates that the patient is still connected to the anaesthetic machine and that there is not an obstruction anywhere.

Respiratory rate

The respiratory rate under anaesthesia should be similar to the resting rate in the conscious animal, although it is often reduced during general anaesthesia especially following induction with barbiturates. An increase in rate usually indicates that the patient is becoming light and a decreased rate usually indicates an increase in level of unconsciousness.

It is important to remember however, that an increased rate may also be seen in a hypoxic animal because they are trying to obtain more oxygen.

Respiratory depth

The depth of respiration is important, and the VN should be able to see good movement of the chest wall and the bag on the anaesthetic circuit, and ensure that the patient is receiving its required tidal volume – 10–15 ml/kg – by checking the minute flow rates. A Wright's respirometer can be used to find out the tidal volume.

Respiratory pattern

The pattern of ventilation during anaesthesia should be regular.

As the level of unconsciousness increases, respiration becomes irregular and the patient may 'gasp' until respiration ceases altogether. The respiration pattern usually becomes irregular and faster if the animal is insufficiently anaesthetised.

CARDIOVASCULAR SYSTEM

Heart rate

It is important that cardiac output is maintained during anaesthesia to ensure adequate perfusion of tissues and vital organs (brain, heart, liver and kidneys). By listening to the heart sounds and feeling a pulse, the VN will be able to detect subtle changes early on and take appropriate steps to maintain cardiac output (e.g. lightening the volatile agent, initiating intravenous fluid therapy). Every anaesthetised animal should have an oesophageal stethoscope placed to facilitate constant heart rate and rhythm monitoring. An electrocardiogram (ECG) can indicate electrical activity and by counting the complexes on the trace, the heart rate can be assessed.

Pulse

The VN must start palpating a pulse at the beginning of anaesthesia and continue regularly throughout the procedure so that subtle changes can be detected. Palpation of the pulse allows the heart rate and the pulse quality to be measured. A strong and easily palpated pulse indicates good pressure and good cardiac output. In contrast, a weak, thready pulse indicates hypotension, hypovolaemia and increase in the level of unconsciousness. It is advisable to palpate a peripheral pulse rather than a central pulse. This is because peripheral pulses are more sensitive to changes in the circulation and therefore changes can be detected earlier.

Peripheral pulse sites:

• Sublingual (ventral-midline surface of the tongue)

- Dorsal pedal artery (caudo-medial surface of hock)
- Digital artery (palmar aspect of the carpus)

Central pulse sites:

- Femoral artery (medial aspect of proximal thigh)

Rhythm

The rhythm of the heart and pulse should be regular and constant. Dysrhythmias may indicate deep levels of unconsciousness and/or hypovolaemia. An ECG is useful to detect cardiac dysrhythmias and heart rate. It is, however, important that the VN is aware that it is possible for an ECG trace to be relatively normal even if the heart muscle is not contracting at all (electromechanical dissociation). For this reason, the VN should not rely on ECG traces alone as monitoring methods.

BLOOD PRESSURE

Arterial blood pressure is monitored by nerve endings in the arterial wall (baroreceptors). These monitor the blood pressure and make changes accordingly (vasoconstriction, vasodilation, increase in heart rate, etc.). During anaesthesia, these responses are depressed. Table 24.1 show normal values for the dog and cat.

Measurement of blood pressure gives a clear indication of the peripheral circulation and can indicate more accurately whether the patient is hypotensive or hypertensive. Maintenance of blood pressure is important so that vital organs are adequately perfused.

A low blood pressure (<mean 60 mmHg) may indicate hypotension. Many anaesthetic drugs cause a dose-dependent fall in blood pressure and this should be taken into consideration.

Blood pressure can be monitored *directly* by arterial cannulation, connected to a pressure transducer or *indirectly* by using an occlusive cuff and Doppler detectors or machine.

Table 24.1 Normal blood pressure in the dog and cat.

Heart response	Blood pressure
Systolic – contraction of the heart	110–160 mmHg
Diastolic – relaxation of the heart	60–100 mmHg

The Doppler device detects an ultrasound echo from the blood passing through the vessel.

MUCOUS MEMBRANES

Observation of the colour of the mucous membranes is extremely useful to assess the condition of the patient's circulation. The mucous membranes should be pink, but as with many other signs, it is important to know the colour that they were *before* the start of anaesthesia so that it is possible to make a comparison.

Pale mucous membranes indicate hypotension/hypovolaemia due to a fall in peripheral perfusion.

Blue (cyanotic) membranes indicate that the patient is being inadequately oxygenated. Remember, however, that the mucous membranes are slow to react to hypoxia and cyanosis is really only ever seen when things are extremely serious and severe.

CAPILLARY REFILL TIME

Capillary refill time (CRT) should be less than 2 seconds. Increased CRT may indicate hypotension, hypovolaemia, toxaemia and/or haemorrhage.

REFLEXES

As the level of unconsciousness deepens, so muscle tone is lost. Some of the following reflexes are useful as a way of assessing the level of unconsciousness but they should always be used in conjunction with other observation methods.

Jaw tone
Not very accurate or sensitive, it is soon lost after induction.

Pedal withdrawal reflex
Not very accurate or sensitive, again it is soon lost after induction.

Palpebral reflex
This is the most useful of all of the reflexes to check. It can be done by *gently* tapping the medial canthus of the eye or by gently brushing the animal's eyelashes. Used in combination

with other signs, it can be used to assess the level of unconsciousness. The reflex is present in conscious animals and it
becomes less apparent during anaesthesia. For most surgical
procedures it is necessary that the palpebral reflex is absent. A
return of the reflex indicates a lightening of the anaesthesia or
an insufficient level of unconsciousness.

Corneal reflex
A corneal reflex is present until very deep anaesthesia (death!)
and should never be used to assess the depth of anaesthesia
because the cornea can be easily damaged.

Pupil diameter
The pupil diameter does increase as the patient becomes more
deeply unconscious. However, it does also depend on some of
the drugs used in premedication regimes (e.g. atropine dilates
the pupil whilst opioid drugs constrict the pupil).

Eye position
The eye rotates down and medially during anaesthesia. If it returns to normal position during anaesthesia, it could indicate
that the animal is becoming too light or too deep. Usually, if
the animal is too light, the eye returns to normal position and
a palpebral reflex is present. If the animal is too deep, the eye
returns to its normal position, but there is no palpebral reflex
and the pupil tends to dilate. This may also be accompanied by
a drying out of the corneal surface and wrinkled appearance.

TEMPERATURE

It is important to obtain a core body temperature before anaesthesia and then regularly throughout and after the procedure.
During anaesthesia, patients inevitably become hypothermic.
This is due to a combination of factors including an anaesthetic
depression of the hypothalamus (decreases temperature reg-
ulation), cold anaesthetic gases, cold theatres, large clipped
areas on the body, cold wet drapes and cold, wet solutions
used cleaning the patient. It is essential to take steps to avoid
hypothermia because it is not only uncomfortable and un-
pleasant for the recovering patient but it can also lead to prolonged recovery times, shock and death. This is particularly
true in small dogs, cats and other small mammals.

ANAESTHESIA

ANAESTHETIC MONITORING AIDS AND EQUIPMENT

As previously stated, *all* anaesthetised animals should have an oesophageal stethoscope placed so that the anaesthetist can listen to the heart and respiratory sounds frequently and if necessary constantly without disturbing the drapes and surgeon. Other monitoring aids such as electrocardiographs, pulse oximeters, respiratory monitors, blood pressure monitors, capnographs (carbon dioxide monitors) are extremely useful in the critical, high-risk patient. However, the most reliable and effective method of assessing levels of unconsciousness is by the anaesthetist physically observing and touching the patient.

Electrocardiogram – measures the electrical activity of the heart. Paper trace monitors are more useful for diagnosing heart rhythm abnormalities whereas the oscilloscope display is more useful for continual monitoring during anaesthesia. The nurse should recognise a normal trace and alert the veterinary surgeon should any abnormalities arise such as dysrhythmia or ectopic beats (an additional heartbeat originating from elsewhere on the heart).

Pulse oximeters – monitor both the pulse rate and the arterial oxygen saturation of the blood. They are placed on the tongue, toe web or ear pinna. The normal value for an animal breathing room air is greater than 95%, but the anaesthetised patient on oxygen should be nearer 100%. Values less than 90% are seriously low indicating inadequate oxygenation of the patient. See Fig. 24.2.

Arterial blood gas analysis – these machines can measure oxygen, carbon dioxide and also the pH of arterial blood. They are very useful for accurately monitoring respiratory function but are very expensive and so not routinely used in most veterinary practices.

Respiratory monitors – have limited value as they indicate that the animal is breathing but give no indication of the tidal volume.

Capnograph – measures the end tidal carbon dioxide (CO_2) content. This approximates to that of arterial blood. A device is placed between the endotracheal tube and the anaesthetic circuit. The normal value for end tidal CO_2 is between 35 and 40 mmHg. Values above 50 mmHg indicate hypercapnia (high levels of CO_2 from hypoventilation).

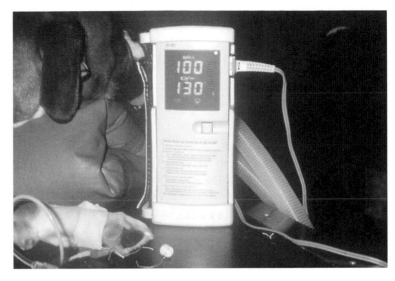

Fig. 24.2 Pulse oximeter

THE QUICK GUIDE TO MONITORING AN ANAESTHETISED ANIMAL

- Watch and monitor the animal *at all times* during the anaesthetic. Do not leave the animal at any time
- Place an oesophageal stethoscope for *every* anaesthetic
- Obtain the following vital signs and at the start and then *at least* every 5 minutes throughout the procedure:
  - Heart rate (see Table 24.2 for normal values)
  - Respiration rate
  - Capillary refill time
  - Pulse quality
- Obtain a core temperature at the start and then at the end of the procedure

Table 24.2 Normal values of vital signs for the anaesthetised dog and cat.

Parameter	Dog	Cat
Heart rate	80–140 bpm	110–140 bpm
Respiration rate	10–30 bpm	20–40 bpm
Temperature	38.3–38.7°C	38–38.5°C
	(100.9–101.7°F)	(100.4–101.6°F)
Capillary refill time	< 2 seconds	< 2 seconds
Oxygen saturation	> 95%	> 95%
Diastolic blood pressure	60–100 mmHg	60–100 mmHg
Systolic blood pressure	110–160 mmHg	110–160 mmHg

- Write down the findings on an anaesthetic chart or piece of paper
- Check the position of the eye (should be rotated ventro-medially)
- Check the palpebral reflex (should be absent during procedure)

THE QUICK GUIDE TO ANAESTHETIC OVERDOSE OR ANIMAL BEING TOO DEEP

- Heart rate: reduced
- Respiration rate: either reduced or panting/gasping
- Pulse quality: rapid, weak, feeble pulse or none detectable
- CRT: >2 seconds
- Colour: pale or cyanotic
- Eye position: up in the normal position
- Palpebral reflex: absent
- Pupil size: dilated
- Temperature: reduced core temperature, animal feels cold to touch
- Surgical wounds: reduced/no haemorrhage present

CHAPTER 25

THE ANAESTHETIC MACHINE

All anaesthetic equipment should be checked regularly for faults. Faulty equipment should be labelled and replaced as soon as possible. It is important that the VN understands the function of the various parts of the anaesthetic machine to ensure they are working correctly.

GAS SUPPLY

GAS CYLINDERS

Inhalation gases are supplied under pressure, in metal cylinders of increasing sizes.

The smaller of these cylinders (sizes AA to E) are mounted directly onto the anaesthetic machine via the pin-index system. The larger cylinders are used to provide piped gases. They are usually stored in a separate room within the building or in an outside lockup.

THE PIN-INDEX SYSTEM

The cylinder valve face has two holes, which correspond to the pins on the machine. The holes for the nitrous oxide and oxygen cylinders are different to ensure the cylinders are not connected to the wrong port.

A BODOC washer ensures a firm seal between cylinder and machine.

CYLINDER COLOUR CODING

All gas cylinders are colour coded:

- Oxygen: black with white top
- Nitrous oxide: blue

- Carbon dioxide: grey

Some older machines have the facility to carry:

- Cyclopropane: orange

Oxygen is supplied as a gas at a pressure of approximately 13300 kPa (1935 psi).

Nitrous oxide is supplied at a pressure of approximately 5100 kPa. At this pressure, nitrous oxide is a liquid. The cylinder contains liquid and some vaporised gas; as the gas is used up more liquid is vaporised.

REDUCING VALVES/REGULATORS

- Reduces the pressure in the cylinder to a lower working pressure
- Maintains constant pressure
- Situated between cylinder and flow meter

PRESSURE/CONTENTS GAUGES

- May be combined with the reducing valve
- O_2 pressure gauge indicates volume of gas remaining in cylinder
- N_2O pressure gauge will remain constant ('full') until the liquid evaporates when the pressure will fall rapidly

FLOW METERS ('ROTAMETER')

- Control the flow of gas indicating in 'litres per minute' (l/min) the quantity passing through the machine and to the patient
- The level is indicated by a 'bobbin' or 'ball' which floats in a calibrated glass tube
- Flow meters should be serviced regularly to check correct readings are given
- The flow rate is taken from the *top* of the *bobbin,* and the *middle* of the *ball bearing*

VAPORISERS

The vaporiser is used to store and administer the volatile anaesthetic agent. It is capable of delivering the volatile agent at various concentrations. The vaporisers must be used with the correct volatile anaesthetic and must not be interchanged. Vaporisers *must* be kept upright at all times to ensure the calibration is correct. See Fig. 25.1.

IN-CIRCUIT VAPORISERS

- Stephens machine or Komasaroff
- The patient's inspiratory efforts draw gas through the vaporiser
- The deeper or more rapid breathing = higher concentration

USING A VAPORISER – IN-CIRCUIT SYSTEM

When using an in-circuit vaporiser (i.e. a Stephen's or Komarosoff machine) remember the following points:

- If anaesthesia is too light – surgical stimulation will lead to an increase in ventilation and therefore a deepening of unconsciousness.

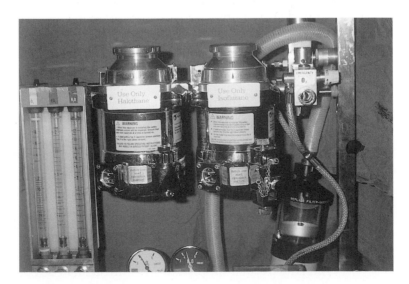

Fig. 25.1 Vaporisers.

- If the vaporiser setting is too high, deepening anaesthesia depresses the ventilation and reduces vaporisation. This acts to some extent as a built in safety factor.
- If the animal stops breathing then no fresh vapour enters the circuit.
- The smaller the fresh gas flow the greater the economy in the use of the volatile agent. (Ensure that oxygen requirements are adequate.)
- A simple, low efficiency vaporiser is required (a Goldman vaporiser for halothane limits the concentration to less than 3%.)
- A sudden increase in ventilation and, therefore of inspired concentration may be dangerous.
- The fact that respired gases pass through the vaporiser introduces the problem of resistance to breathing.

OXYGEN FLUSH

Also known as 'purge' or 'bypass' valve. Oxygen bypasses the vaporiser and exits through the common gas outlet.
Used for:

- Emergency resuscitation
- Flushing the anaesthetic from the circuit before patient disconnection

WARNING DEVICES

Some machines are fitted with warning devices to indicate a lack of oxygen supply. This is obviously a huge advantage. Without doubt there have been many anaesthetic deaths or near-deaths through there being no alarm system and animals receiving either no oxygen supply or a lethal supply of nitrous oxide and halothane. When purchasing a new machine, always check that there is an oxygen alarm device.

There are two main types:

THE BOSUN WHISTLE

This alarm is dependent on there being a flow of nitrous oxide. When the oxygen supply fails the nitrous will be cut off and a whistle will sound. Newer machines have alarms that depend on only the falling oxygen supply.

OVER-PRESSURE ALARM

High pressure that may occur when circuit valves are left closed will sound an alarm. This alarm may be tested by occluding the common outlet valve whilst depressing the oxygen flush button.

CARBON DIOXIDE ABSORBERS

Rebreathing systems incorporate a carbon dioxide absorbent, which consists of:

- Sodium hydroxide ('soda')
- Calcium hydroxide ('lime')
- Silicates
- A pH indicator
- Colour change: pink to white or white to lilac

The colour change indicates that the absorbent is exhausted and should be changed. It is important also to be aware that some absorbents change back to the original colour if left overnight.

CHANGING THE ABSORBENT

Soda lime is an irritant alkaline substance. The dust must not be inhaled or allowed in contact with the eyes. Wear gloves and a facemask with protective eye goggles.

CHECKING AND SETTING UP THE ANAESTHETIC MACHINE

The anaesthetic machine must be thoroughly checked at the beginning of each day:

(1) Connect and switch on scavenging system
(2) Check the vaporiser is full (should be filled the night before) and that the dial can be moved easily
(3) Check that all of the cylinders are full
(4) Check that piped gas supply is switched on (where applicable)

(5) Check that the flow meters work

(6) Check warning devices work

(7) Check emergency oxygen flush works

At the end of the day:

(1) Fill the vaporiser in a well ventilated room

(2) Replace empty cylinders

(3) Switch cylinders off and empty system of remaining gas

(4) Clean and disinfect all surfaces

CHAPTER 26

ANAESTHETIC SYSTEMS

Inhalation anaesthetic agents may be administered via anaesthetic systems. During the early days of veterinary anaesthesia, a liquid anaesthetic agent (ether, chloroform, trichloroethylene) would be applied to a gauze swab and applied either directly to the patient's nose or placed into a face mask. These were called 'open' and 'semiopen' methods of administering inhalation anaesthesia. The disadvantages of these methods include high pollution risks, little control over 'depth' of anaesthesia and dangerous fluctuations in levels of anaesthesia.

Later on, apparatus was developed that provided a link between an anaesthetic machine and an intubated patient. These systems provided a route for the administration of anaesthetic gases and for the removal of expired carbon dioxide (CO_2).

There are various methods by which anaesthetic systems are classified (American and UK writers have different definitions of 'closed' and 'semiclosed' systems and then there are the Mapleson classifications). It's a good idea to be aware of the various terms, however. Hall and Clarke (1991) suggest that the most clinically useful method of categorising the different systems is based on the method by which carbon dioxide is removed from the circuit.

• Nonrebreathing systems (semiclosed)

and

• Rebreathing systems (closed)

Nonrebreathing systems rely on a high fresh gas flow to vent expired gases out of the system into the atmosphere whilst rebreathing systems pass the expired gases through a canister containing soda lime which removes the carbon dioxide and allows the same gas to be rebreathed by the patient.

NONREBREATHING SYSTEMS

- Ayre's T-piece
- Magill
- Lack (coaxial and parallel)
- Bain

These systems work by providing a fresh gas flow rate, which is pooled into a reservoir from which the patient inhales the fresh gas and volatile agent combination. Expired gas from the patient is also passed into this area and then out into the atmosphere via a spill valve. For this reason, it is important that the fresh gas flow rates are high enough to help push out the exhaled CO_2-rich gas and provide enough for the next inspiration. It is important that the patient's respiratory tidal and minute volume is calculated and the gas settings fixed appropriately depending on the circuit used. Table 26.1 outlines the advantages and disadvantages of nonrebreathing systems.

METHOD OF CALCULATING RESPIRATORY MINUTE VOLUME

$$\text{minute volume} = \text{body weight (kg)} \times 10\text{–}15\,\text{ml} \times \text{respiratory rate}/\text{minute}$$

Minute volume must then be multiplied by the anaesthetic system factor (see notes on individual systems).

Table 26.1   Advantages and disadvantages of nonrebreathing systems.

Advantages	Disadvantages
Less resistance than with rebreathing systems	High gas flow rates required to prevent rebreathing of expired gases
Less expensive to purchase than rebreathing systems	High atmospheric pollution hazard
The concentration of anaesthetic can be changed rapidly	Higher consumption rate of the volatile agent used
Known quantities of gases can be administered, inspired quantity is similar to the amount set on the dial	Dry and cold inspiratory gases causing an increased risk of patient hypothermia
De-nitrogenation is not required during initial connection to the patient	Increased running costs because of high gas flows required
Nitrous oxide can be administered safely	

AYRE'S T-PIECE (MAPLESON 'E' AND 'F')

There are no valves in this system, which means there is very little resistance to breathing, thereby making it the most suitable system for very small animals. As a general guide, this would be any animal weighing under 10 kg. Usually, the T-piece is fitted with an open-ended bag on the distal end of the system. This is called the *Jackson-Rees modification* and enables intermittent positive pressure ventilation (IPPV) and can be used as a method of monitoring respiration.

Fresh gas passes along the narrow tubing from the anaesthetic machine towards the patient. Some of this gas passes into the corrugated tubing so that when the patient inhales it takes most of its gas supply from this area. Exhaled gases from the patient are also forced into this part of the system by the continuing fresh gas coming down tube. During the patient's expiratory pause, the exhaled gas is pushed out of the system via the bag, and a fresh supply of gas is collected in ready for the patient's next inhalation. Relatively high fresh gas flow rates of 2.5–3 multiplied by the minute volume are required to prevent rebreathing. The main disadvantages of this system are the high gas flow rates required and the difficulty in scavenging waste anaesthetic gases.

The main advantages of the T-piece are that effective IPPV can be carried out and its suitability for very small animals due to the low resistance of the system.

Mapleson 'E' classification refers to the system without the Jackson-Rees modification, Mapleson 'F' describes the addition of the bag. See Fig. 26.1 for Ayre's T-piece.

MAGILL (MAPLESON 'A')

The patient inhales fresh gas from the wide-bore corrugated tubing and reservoir bag, which is on the proximal end of the system. Some of the exhaled gases pass back up this tubing, but during the expiratory pause, the continuous fresh gas flow forces the last part of the expired gas (rich in CO_2) out through a Heidebrink valve into the atmosphere. A flow rate of at least the same as or slightly more than the patient's minute volume is required to prevent rebreathing. There is slight resistance to breathing due to the presence of the valve and this makes this system unsuitable for use in animals less than 5 kg. There is no upper weight limit for this system. The

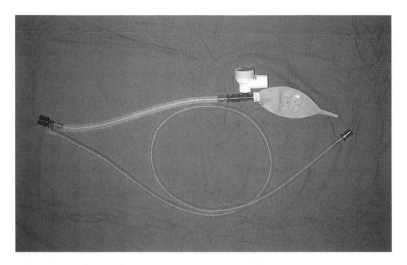

Fig. 26.1   Ayre's T-piece.

main disadvantage of this system is that it is not satisfactory for prolonged positive-pressure ventilation (expired gas is forced back into the lungs when the bag is squeezed instead of being removed via the expiratory valve, resulting in patient hypercapnia and hypoxia). The valve is situated on the distal end of the circuit making the circuit clumsy when used during head surgery.

LACK (MODIFIED MAPLESON 'A')

This is available as a coaxial or parallel system. Coaxial simply means one tube inside the other. These systems were developed to help control atmospheric pollution. The expiratory valve is placed at the anaesthetic machine end of the system, which facilitates easier scavenging of waste gases. Fresh anaesthetic gases pass down the outer corrugated tube to the patient, and in a similar way to the Magill, some of the expired gases pass back up this tube. During the respiratory pause, the fresh gas supply pushes the last part of expired gas out of the valve via the inner expiratory tube.

The position of the valve at the anaesthetic machine end of the system facilitates surgery on the head and makes this a less bulky system than the Magill. The Lack is not suitable for prolonged positive-pressure ventilation. A flow rate of 1–1.5 multiplied by the minute volume is recommended to prevent

rebreathing. See Fig. 26.2 Coaxial Lack, and Fig. 26.3 Parallel
Lack.

BAIN – MODIFIED MAPLESON 'D'

Externally, the Bain looks almost identical to the coaxial Lack,
however, this system works very differently and functions in

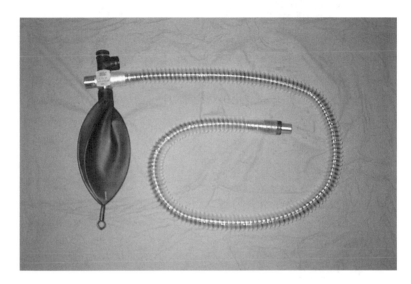

Fig. 26.2 Coaxial Lack.

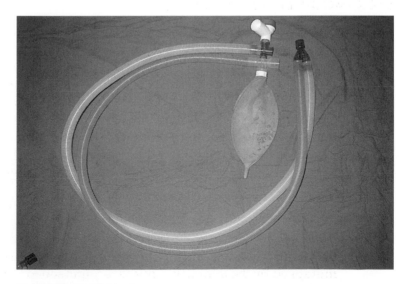

Fig. 26.3 Parallel Lack.

a similar way to the T-piece. Fresh gas passes along the thin inner tube to the patient and expired gas through the outer sleeve to the bag and valve, which are placed on the machine end of the system. Just like the T-piece, high gas flow rates are required to prevent significant rebreathing of expired gas. This is suitable for patients over 10 kg.

The main disadvantage of this system is that very high gas flow rates are required, especially in heavier dogs, and so effective scavenging is essential. Also, coaxial systems present an operational risk if the inner tube becomes detached because very large dead space is created. This should be checked on a regular basis by occluding the patient end and passing 6 l/min of oxygen through the tubing. If there are no leaks in the system, the oxygen bobbin will dip and the machine pressure relief valve will be activated. A flow rate of 2.5–3 multiplied by the minute volume should be used in this system to prevent rebreathing. See Fig. 26.4.

REBREATHING SYSTEMS

- Circle
- To and fro

These systems work in a completely different way to the non-rebreathing systems and as their name suggests, exhaled gas

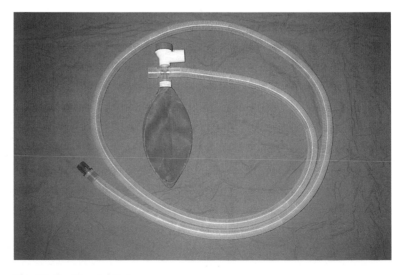

Fig. 26.4 Coaxial Bain.

is rebreathed after passing through a canister of soda lime granules (90% calcium hydroxide, 5% sodium hydroxide and 5% silicate), which remove the carbon dioxide. These systems use far less anaesthetic gas and volatile agent and produce less atmospheric pollution. These systems can be run completely closed at very low flow rates or slightly higher gas flow rates can be used and excess gas is passed out into the atmosphere via an overflow valve. These systems have high resistance because of the packed soda lime and should only be used in animals over 10 kg. They are the most suitable and economic systems for use in large animal anaesthesia. Frequent observation of the colour of the soda lime granules is necessary to assess if they have become exhausted. It must be noted that colour change is no guarantee that the soda lime is not exhausted. A more accurate assessment can be made by wrapping a small quantity in some gauze and blowing over it. The soda lime should heat up. If it does not it indicates that the soda lime is exhausted. The VN must also be aware that different makes of soda lime have different colour changes from fresh to exhausted, e.g. pink to white or white to pink. Nitrous oxide should not be used with these systems unless an oxygen meter/pulse oximeter is used throughout the anaesthetic. This is due to the high concentration of nitrous oxide in the exhaled gas building up in the system and resulting in patient hypoxia. There are two important factors to be aware of when using rebreathing systems: following connection the concentration of the volatile agent is greatly reduced because it is mixed with the exhaled gas. Equilibrium occurs as soon as a certain blood concentration of anaesthetic gases has been reached, and gaseous agents are then exhaled from the body relatively unchanged. This first mixture of exhaled gas also contains nitrogen and this decreases the oxygen concentration of inhaled gas. To overcome these problems, the circle and to and fro are best run as a nonrebreathing systems until the patient is at the required level of anaesthesia. This means increasing the flow rate and opening the overspill valve.

It should also be remembered that during anaesthesia, the concentration of volatile agent within the system will progressively increase and the amount the patient inhales will not resemble what is dialled on the vaporiser. The oxygen consumption in the dog is 4–5 ml/kg/min. In theory this is all that is required to be set when using a to and fro or circle system, however, due to nitrogen build up in the system, a flow rate of 0.5–2 l/min is advisable.

As a general rule, it is advisable always to use these systems with the valve open, and not to use them as totally closed circuits. For the first 5–10 minutes, run them at about 3 litres and then reduce to 1 litre for the remainder of the anaesthetic time. (Table 26.2 outlines the advantages and disadvantages of rebreathing systems.)

TO AND FRO SYSTEM

The disadvantages of this circuit far outweigh the benefits and they include:

- Cumbersome apparatus near the patient's head, may get in the way of surgery and can become disconnected from the ET tube or the patient may become extubated
- The dead space increases throughout anaesthesia as the soda lime nearest the patient gets exhausted
- The soda lime canister is very close to the patient's airway and there is a high risk of the irritant granules being inhaled and causing bronchitis
- The soda lime granules heat up as a result of absorbing the exhaled carbon dioxide and this can cause hyperthermia
- The canisters are positioned horizontally and unless the canisters are packed tightly, rebreathing of CO_2 can occur as exhaled gas passes over the top of the granules or channels form through the soda lime

Table 26.2 Advantages and disadvantages of rebreathing systems

Advantages	Disadvantages
Low gas flow rates – cheaper running costs	Soda lime canister causes a high resistance to breathing
Less atmospheric pollution	Depth of anaesthesia is slow to change
Less volatile anaesthetic agent used	Denitrogenation is required during initial connection
Expired heat and vapour are conserved in the circuit – less risk of hypothermia	Expensive to purchase
	Risk of rebreathing of CO_2-rich expired gases if soda lime exhausted
	Inspired gas and volatile agent concentration is unknown – nitrous oxide must be used with great care can lead to hypoxia
	Only suitable for animals over 10 kg in weight

THE CIRCLE SYSTEM

This system has far fewer of the problems of the to and fro system. The soda lime canister is placed in the vertical position far away from the patient's head. This means that soda lime inhalation, hyperthermia and an increase in dead space throughout anaesthesia are avoided. The inspiratory and expiratory tubes are fitted with unidirectional valves to ensure that the gases pass only in one direction. The main disadvantage of this system is that the combination of soda lime canister and the valves make this a high resistance system suitable only for animals over 10 kg.

FURTHER READING

Hall, L.W. and Clarke, K.W. (1991) *Veterinary Anaesthesia*. Bailliere Tindall, London.

McKelvey, D. and Hollingshead, K.W. (1994) *Mosby's Fundamentals of Veterinary Technology, Small Animal Anaesthesia Canine and Feline Practice.* Mosby, USA.

SECTION 5
RADIOGRAPHY

CHAPTER 27

PRACTICAL RADIOGRAPHY

INTRODUCTION

The VN should be able to produce radiographs of diagnostic quality and in order to do this, should have an understanding of the processes involved in producing the radiograph. This should also include understanding the dangers of ionising radiation and being able to take adequate precautions.

This section deals with the practical side of radiography, positioning the animal, processing the radiograph and assisting with contrast radiography. In order to carry this out safely the nurse should understand the dangers of radiography.

IONISING RADIATION

The potential dangers of radiation are often underestimated because:

- They are invisible
- They are painless
- Their effects are latent (may take years to become apparent)
- Effects are cumulative – repeated low doses have an additive effect.

EFFECTS OF RADIATION INJURY

Radiation damages living tissues by changing biological molecules. Even low doses can cause cell damage because of the effect of radiation on DNA.

Somatic damage and carcinogenic effects
Damage that occurs to the body during the recipient's lifetime is called somatic damage. Direct changes in the body tissues, such as erythema, alopecia, digestive upsets and pain may

occur soon after exposure although latent affects may not be seen until many years later. Such disorders include cancer, cataracts, sterility and leukaemia.

Genetic damage

Damage can also occur to the reproductive cells, which can cause genetic mutations. These changes to the chromosomal material in the reproductive cells produce changes that are not apparent until future generations are born.

GENERAL SAFETY MEASURES

1. DISTANCE

The intensity of radiation decreases with distance in accordance with the inverse square law. Never be any closer to the primary beam than 2 metres.

2. GOOD RADIOGRAPHIC TECHNIQUE

These steps will help to reduce risks:

- No part of any personnel should ever be within the primary beam
- Collimate to the area of interest
- Use fast film/screen combinations when possible to reduce exposure
- Avoid repeat exposures by using good positioning methods, exposure charts and standardised processing techniques
- Avoid using a grid if not necessary as this will require a higher exposure
- Use positioning aids/anaesthesia to avoid holding animals

3. PREMISES

- Identify the controlled area (2 metres around the primary beam)
- Fifteen centimetre (6′) concrete walls or double-brick
- Lead ply or barium plaster
- Lead screens
- Lead backed table
- Warning notices/lights (lit when exposure taken)

- International radiation symbol displayed on entry to the room

4. EQUIPMENT

- Machines need to be checked and serviced regularly
- Check the accuracy of the light beam diaphragm
- Check the integrity of lead aprons, gloves and screens

5. STAFF

- Limited access to controlled area
- Only essential personnel in the controlled area
- Only trained personnel in the controlled area
- No one under 16 years old in the controlled area
- No pregnant women in the controlled area
- Limited access to controlled area by 16–18 year-old personnel
- Monitor personnel using dosimeters

6. PROTECTIVE CLOTHING

Lead clothing protects against scatter but not against primary radiation:

- Lead aprons (> 0.25 mm lead)
- Lead gloves and hand shields (> 0.35 mm lead)
- Lead thyroid shields
- Lead glasses (ocular tissue is one of the most delicate areas subjected to radiation exposure, yet the eyes are most frequently neglected)

Ensure the equipment is stored correctly and not folded.

CHAPTER 28

SELECTION OF EXPOSURE FACTORS

The exposure factors that are selected have a huge impact on how the finished film will turn out. Generally, the kilovoltage (kV) should be increased as tissue thickness and density increases. The milliamperage (mA) is usually left the same.

Provided that processing techniques are adequate:

- Dark images are over-penetrated – the kV should be reduced
- White, pale images are under-penetrated so the kV should be increased

KILOVOLTAGE (kV)

Increasing the kV will increase the penetrating ability of the X-ray photons and therefore the effect on the film is to produce blacker images of lower contrast. (Contrast is the difference between the white areas and the black areas – high contrast means there are definite areas of black and white and all the greys in between. Low contrast means that there is a general all over greyness.)

MILLIAMPERAGE (mA) AND TIME (s)

The amount of X-rays produced multiplied by the time gives us the milliampere-seconds (mAs). Increasing mAs will produce more X-ray photons. Changing the mAs does not affect the penetrating power of the X-ray photons but it will produce a blacker image on the areas of film that have been penetrated. The relationship between the mA and the seconds allows a range of exposures to be used depending on the machine.

DISTANCE (FILM–FOCAL DISTANCE – FFD)

The distance between the focal spot (in the tube head) and the film affects the quantity of X-rays reaching the film. The greater the distance is, the more the beam spreads out therefore fewer X-rays reach the film. Usually the FFD is kept constant, between 75 cm and 100 cm. (A less powerful machine would require a shorter distance.) If the FFD is increased, the intensity of the beam decreases according to the inverse square law.

> The intensity of the beam is *inversely* proportional to the *square* of the distance from the source.

Therefore if the X-ray tube head is too far away from the object being radiographed, the image will be overly faint or nonexistent.

EXPOSURE CHARTS

An exposure chart provides a quick, visual display of all of the exposures that are needed for each body area. The aim of an exposure chart is to avoid repeating exposures, to save time and wasted films and to reduce the radiation hazard to staff.

Settings can be chosen by assessing the size of the patient, i.e. cat, small dog, medium dog and large dog. See Table 28.1. Be aware that charts apply only to a particular X-ray machine, using constant FFDs, cassettes, films, grid and processing technique.

Table 28.1 Example of a radiographic exposure chart for dogs and cats.

Species and size	Area	mA	kV	Time (s)	FFD	Film	Grid
Dog							
• Giant	Lateral Stifle	100	90	0.6	75 cm	Fuji G8 18 × 24	Yes
• Large	Lateral Stifle	100	85	0.2	75 cm	Fuji G8 18 × 24	No
• Medium	Lateral Stifle	100	80	0.08	75 cm	Fuji G8 18 × 24	No
• Small	Lateral Stifle	100	65	0.02	75 cm	Fuji G8 18 × 24	No
Cat	Lateral Stifle	100	60	0.02	75 cm	Fuji G8 18 × 24	No

OTHER FACTORS TO CONSIDER WHEN SELECTING EXPOSURE SETTINGS

Other factors that should be taken into account when setting the exposure are:

- Movement: as short a time as possible should be selected
- Dressings and casts: the kV must be increased by 10 for casts

Variations from the exposure chart are sometimes necessary because of the limitations of the machinery, limitations of the environment or limitations created by the patient.

Exposure calculations
Film focal distance and the inverse square law
Occasionally, it may be necessary to alter the FFD. For example, if there is a low output X-ray machine, and it is necessary to penetrate thicker tissue than the machine at its usual FFD is capable of (e.g. large animal radiography), it is possible to decrease the FFD in order to achieve penetration and a radiograph of reasonable quality.

   If the FFD is altered, the new exposure can be worked out using this calculation:

$$\text{New mAs} = \text{New FFD}^2 \div \text{Old FFD}^2 \times \text{Old mAs}$$

Example:
   Having been using an exposure of 10 mAs and FFD of 50 cm, what exposure is required if the FFD is changed to 100 cm?

   Answer: $10 \times 10000 \div 2500 = 10 \times 4 = 40$ mAs.

The 10 kV rule
Increasing the kV by 10, does the same (more or less) to the image as doubling the mAs. To put another way, doubling the mAs does the same to the image as increasing the kV by 10. By implication, decreasing the kV by 10 does the same to the image as halving the mAs.

   Why is this useful?

   It is possible to use this rule in all kinds of situations when the machine or patient is causing problems.

For example, the patient is panting and the rapid breathing movement is creating a very badly blurred image on the finished radiograph. The exposure itself was fine, but it is necessary to reduce the exposure *time* to prevent the movement blur.

The first exposure was kV = 80, mAs = 15;
the next exposure is kV = 90, mAs = 7.5.

Another situation where this calculation would be useful is when a darker image is required but the kV is cranked up as high as it will go. By using the 10 rule to keep the kV as it is but doubling the mAs gives the darkening required.

The first exposure was kV = 80, mAs = 15;
the next exposure is kV = 80, mAs = 30.

If the image should stay the same, but it is necessary to jiggle the exposures around, the 10 kV rule works like this:

50 kV at 32 mAs will create the same exposure as:
60 kV at 16 mAs and
70 kV at 8 mAs

So, if an exposure at 20 mAs at 80 kV is adequate, what is the kV required if the mAs are changed to 10?

Answer: The mAs are halved therefore increase kV by 10 = 90 kV.

Milliamperage (mA) and time (s)
This has already been covered in these notes, but as a reminder:

$$mAs = mA \times s$$

If mA is doubled, the time may be halved (thereby decreasing exposure time and reducing the possibility of movement blur).

GRID FACTOR

Grids are used to improve the quality of the finished radiography when radiographing through thicker body parts. When using a grid it is necessary to increase the exposure by something called the *grid factor*:

$$mAs \times grid\ factor\ (GF) = exposure\ required\ using\ grid$$

For example: the exposure factors required for a lateral radiograph of a dog's abdomen might be 3.2 mAs at 80 kV.

If a grid with a grid factor of 3 is used, the new exposure will be 3.2 × 3 = 9.6 mAs at 80 kV.

This may be rather too much time and so the 10 kV rule can be used. By increasing the kV by 10 it is possible to halve the mAs, giving a setting of 90 kV at 4.8 mAs.

CHAPTER 29

RADIOGRAPHIC POSITIONING

The VN should be able to position an animal correctly in order to produce a diagnostic radiograph of any part of the animal. To describe a radiographic projection, the point of entry of the beam is first described followed by the point of exit.

For example, dorso-ventral thorax means that the animal is in sternal recumbency and the X-ray beam enters dorsally through the spine and exits ventrally though the sternum.

The following are terms used to describe radiographic projections.

- Cranial
- Caudal
- Rostral
- Dorsal
- Ventral
- Proximal
- Distal
- Medial
- Lateral
- Palmar
- Plantar

The terms *anterior* (towards the head) and *posterior* (towards the tail) are sometimes used instead of cranial and caudal. See Fig. 29.1.

RESTRAINT

Effective restraint is necessary not only to prevent the animal from moving, but also to help position the area being radiographed so that the best possible view can be achieved.

Restraint can be achieved in two ways:

- Chemically: sedation or general anaesthesia

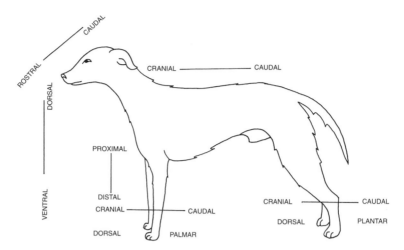

Fig. 29.1   Anatomical directions.

- Positioning aids: ties, sandbags, foam wedges, radiolucent troughs, Velcro™

An animal must *never* be held during radiography. Manual restraint is exceedingly dangerous and should only ever be used in exceptional circumstances. In which case, the requesting VS should restrain the animal. The VN must *never* do this. Under the 1999 Ionising Radiation Regulations it is totally unacceptable to hold animals.

Never use ties to secure body areas on conscious or sedated animals. Serious damage and distress can occur if they are roused and try to move.

ANATOMICAL KNOWLEDGE

Thorough knowledge of anatomy and bony landmarks is essential to ensure good positioning of the animal for radiography. The VN must be fully competent in this, not only for written and practical examinations but also for the following reasons:

- Ensures that all of the relevant area is on the radiograph
- Enables ease of interpretation of the final radiograph
- Standardises methods so that comparisons with books and other radiographs can be made
- Helps to prevent repeat radiographs being taken (safety, cost and time considerations)

- Prevents other body structures obscuring the relevant area
- Structures are not distorted by incorrect centring

POSITIONING OF THE ANIMAL

Being able to produce consistently good radiographs is highly rewarding and an invaluable aid to the VS in the diagnosis of many conditions. To achieve this, it is necessary to standardise patient positioning, centring points and collimation areas. What follows illustrates the main positioning, centring points and collimation areas for most standard radiographic procedures. These are guidelines designed to help the VN in practice and also in examinations. It is important to remember that each case is different and the personal preferences of each VS should be considered.

THORAX

Take the exposure during peak inspiration so that the lungs are fully expanded and aerated. This helps to increase the contrast on the finished radiograph.

Keep exposure *time* to a minimum to help reduce movement blur on the finished radiograph.

Lateral

- Place the animal in right or left lateral recumbency
- Extend the forelimbs cranially, secure with sandbags (or ties if anaesthetised)
- Extend the neck and secure with sandbag if necessary
- Place a foam wedge under sternum to help ensure sternum and spine are in the same horizontal plane. See Fig. 29.2.
- Centre on: caudal aspect of the scapula, midway between dorsal edge of scapula and sternum
- Collimate to: (a) manubrium and last rib and (b) lateral skin surfaces

Dorso-ventral

- Sternal recumbency
- Forelimbs extended cranially, secured with sandbags or ties
- Sandbags either side of animal to help prevent lateral rotation of the body. See Fig. 29.3.

RADIOGRAPHY

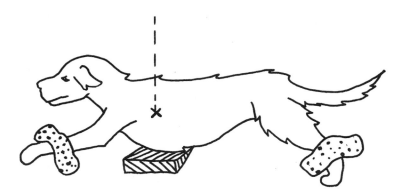

Fig. 29.2   Thorax lateral view.

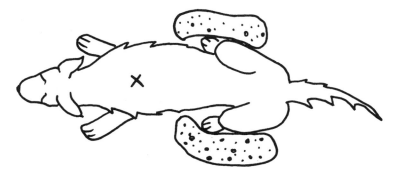

Fig. 29.3   Thorax dorso-ventral view.

- Centre on: midline at the level of the caudal scapula
- Collimate to: (a) manubrium and last rib and (b) lateral skin surfaces

Ventro-dorsal
This view is rarely carried out because the heart adopts a more natural position during dorso-ventral (DV) views and as described below, it is potentially dangerous for dyspnoeic animals to be positioned for this view.

- Dorsal recumbency
- Forelimbs extended cranially, secured with sandbags or ties
- Sandbags or trough to prevent lateral rotation of the body. See Fig. 29.4.
- Centre on: midline at the level of the caudal scapula

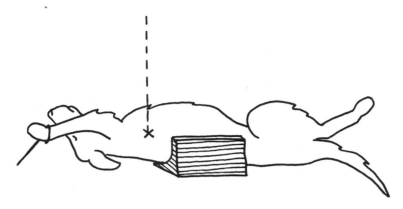

Fig. 29.4   Thorax ventro-dorsal view.

- Collimate to: (a) manubrium and last rib and (b) lateral skin surfaces

Note: Avoid placing a dyspnoeic animal in dorsal recumbency for a ventro-dorsal view of the thorax as this can exacerbate the problem. This particularly applies to an animal with a ruptured diaphragm.

ABDOMEN

It is usually recommended that the animal be starved for at least 12 hours prior to abdominal radiography.

Cleaning and brushing and drying the coat first will help to produce clearer pictures by removing confusing radiodensities.

It is advisable to administer an enema before any radiographic studies of the uro-genital tract and colon.

Take exposure during expiration

Centring and collimation of the primary beam has been described below for general abdominal views. If specific organs and structures are required, centring of the primary beam will need to be altered to take this into consideration.

For example, the beam will need to be centred further cranially for examinations of the liver. Bladder studies will require that the beam be centred further caudal. Good anatomical knowledge is required to be able to perform the required task appropriately.

RADIOGRAPHY

Lateral

- Animal in lateral recumbency (usually right lateral recumbency – be consistent)
- Hind limbs extended caudally and secured with sandbags or ties
- A foam wedge may be placed between the stifles and under the sternum to help reduce horizontal rotation of the body. See Fig. 29.5.
- Centre on: last rib, midway between dorsal and ventral skin surface (for general abdominal view).
- Collimate to: (a) just cranial to the xiphisternum and to the greater trochanter and (b) the spine dorsally and the ventral skin surface

Ventro-dorsal

- Animal in dorsal recumbency
- Sandbags or troughs to prevent lateral rotation of the body
- Hind limbs extended caudally. See Fig. 29.6.
- Centre on: midline, level with the last rib
- Collimate to: (a) just cranial to the xiphisternum and to the greater trochanter and (b) the lateral skin edges

The dorso-ventral views of the abdomen are rarely indicated. Exceptions would be for dyspnoeic patients and those having contrast studies of the stomach.

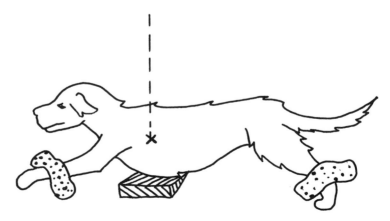

Fig. 29.5   Abdomen lateral view.

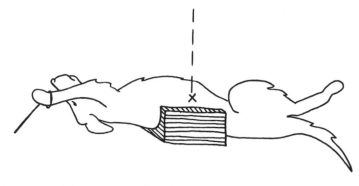

Fig. 29.6   Abdomen ventro-dorsal view.

RADIOGRAPHY

SKULL

Anaesthesia is required for all views of the skull to enable good positioning. If present the endotracheal tube should be temporarily removed during exposure, to avoid confusing artefacts on the finished radiograph.

The views described below demonstrate the positioning, centring and collimation for general views of the skull. This may vary depending on the area of interest and good anatomical knowledge of the skull is required to obtain relevant radiographs.

Lateral

- Animal in lateral recumbency
- Place small foam wedge under the muzzle to ensure that the sagittal plane of the skull is parallel to the cassette
- Extend neck. See Fig. 29.7.
- Centre: midway between the eye and the ear
- Collimate to: (a) external nares to caudal skull and (b) dorsal and ventral skin surfaces

Dorso-ventral

- Animal in sternal recumbency, neck extended
- Place head and cassette on a foam block or other, to make sure entire skull is parallel to the cassette
- Place sandbag over neck to help prevent lateral rotation. See Fig. 29.8.
- Centre on: midline, level with the medial canthus of the eye

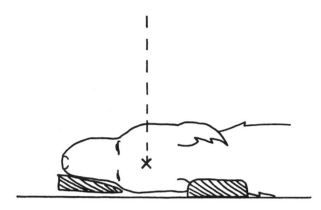

Fig. 29.7   Skull lateral view.

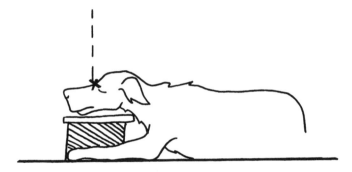

Fig. 29.8   Skull dorso-ventral view.

- Collimate to: (a) external nares to caudal skull and (b) dorsal and ventral skin surfaces

Ventro-dorsal

- Animal in trough in dorsal recumbency, neck extended
- Place foam pad under the neck to help ensure palate is parallel to the cassette
- Place adhesive tape around the upper canines and fixed to the table top or cassette. See Fig. 29.9.
- Centre on: midline, level with the medial canthus of the eye
- Collimate to: as dorso-ventral view

Rostro-caudal

This view is performed to evaluate the frontal sinuses, temporal area and zygomatic arch. An 'open-mouth' rostro-caudal view is obtained mainly to evaluate the tympanic bullae.

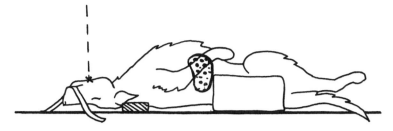

Fig. 29.9   Skull ventro-dorsal view.

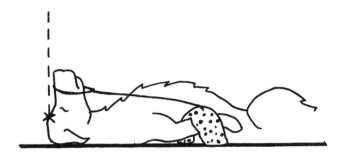

Fig. 29.10   Skull rostro-caudal view.

- Animal in trough in dorsal recumbency
- Limbs secured caudally using sandbags to help prevent lateral rotation
- Ties applied around the muzzle so that the skull is perpendicular to the cassette. See Fig. 29.10.

Open-mouth rostro-caudal

As before, placing a tie around maxilla and secured to the table to ensure skull and hard palate are perpendicular to the cassette.

Pull the mouth open and place a tie around the mandible and secure to the table. Pull the tongue out of the mouth as much as possible. See Fig. 29.11.

- Direct primary beam at a 5–10° angle to the vertical.
- Centre on: midline, between the eyes (bulla – midline, base of the tongue)
- Collimate to: the skin surfaces around the skull

Intra-oral

This view is used chiefly to evaluate the teeth and nasal cavity.

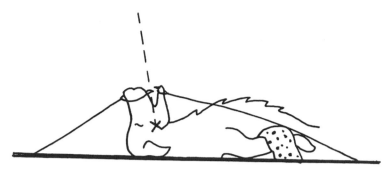

Fig. 29.11   Skull open-mouth rostro-caudal view.

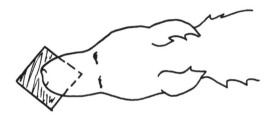

Fig. 29.12   Skull intra-oral view.

- Animal in sternal recumbency
- Troughs or sandbags to prevent lateral rotation
- Muzzle placed on a foam block
- Cassette or nonscreen film placed in the mouth over the tongue. See Fig. 29.12.
- Centre on: depends on the area of interest but generally, midline halfway along muzzle
- Collimate to: include nasal chambers from the external nares to caudal oral cavity

VERTEBRAL COLUMN

Lateral spine
Patient in lateral recumbency

- Foam pads placed under mandible, cervical and lumbar spine to help ensure that the spine is parallel to the table-top
- Foam wedge under sternum and in between legs to help prevent rotation of the body
- Forelimbs drawn caudally and secured. See Figs 29.13 and 29.14

- Centre on: see below for each vertebral section
- Collimate to: see below for each vertebral section

Ventro-dorsal vertebral column

Ventro-dorsal views of the vertebral column are used in preference to dorso-ventral views to minimise magnification of the vertebral column on the finished radiograph.

- Animal placed into a trough in dorsal recumbency. See Fig. 29.15
- Centre on: along the midline, at points described above depending on the area of interest
- Collimate to: as above and several centimetres lateral to the vertebral column depending on the size of the animal

RADIOGRAPHY

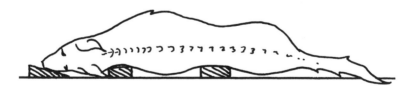

Fig. 29.13 Vertebral column lateral spine view.

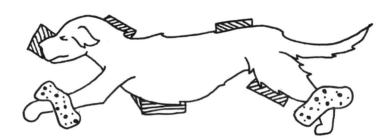

Fig. 29.14 Vertebral column lateral spine view.

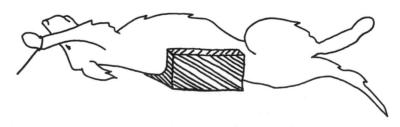

Fig. 29.15 Ventro-dorsal vertebral column view.

1. Cervical spine

- Centre on: midway between the occipital crest and the caudal aspect of the scapula
- Collimate to: (a) occipital crest and caudal aspect of the scapula and (b) dorso-ventrally to include muscle mass but not fat and skin

2. Thoracic spine

- Centre on: level with the caudal aspect of the scapula over the vertebrae (can not be palpated but approximately a couple of centimetre ventral to dorsal skin surface)
- Collimate to: (a) cranial scapula to the last rib and (b) the skin surface caudally

3. Thoraco-lumbar spine

- Centre on: the thoraco-lumbar junction
- Collimate to: (a) three vertebrae cranial and caudal to the thoraco-lumbar junction and (b) the skin surface caudally

4. Lumbar spine

- Centre: midway between the thoraco-lumbar junction and the iliac crest and over transverse spinous processes
- Collimate to: (a) thoraco-lumbar junction and iliac crest and (b) dorsal skin suface

5. Sacral spine

- Centre on: midway between the iliac crest and the greater trochanter
- Collimate to: (a) iliac crest and greater trochanter and (b) dorsal skin surface

PELVIS

Lateral

- Patient in lateral recumbency
- Foam wedges between stifles and under sternum to prevent rotation of the body. See Fig. 29.16
- Centre on: the greater trochanter

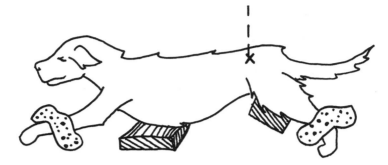

Fig. 29.16 Pelvis lateral view.

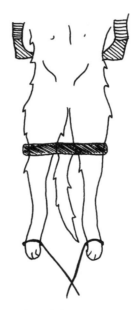

Fig. 29.17 Pelvis ventro-dorsal view.

- Collimate to: (a) the iliac crest and ischial tuberosity and (b) the dorsal skin surface

Ventro-dorsal

- Patient in trough, in dorsal recumbency
- Hindlimbs extended caudally and fixed with ties to the table
- Legs rotated medially to ensure femurs parallel to each other
- Palpate the patellae to ensure they are pointing upwards.
- Secure in the correct position around femurs with adhesive tape or 'Velcro'. See Fig. 29.17

- Centre on: midline, level with the greater trochanters
- Collimate to: (a) iliac crest and patellae and (b) skin surfaces

The patella must be included in the finished radiograph when being submitted for BVA/KC hip score.

FORELIMBS

SHOULDER

Lateral

- Animal in lateral recumbency on the same side as the shoulder being radiographed
- Extend the required limb cranially and secure with tie
- Draw the other limb caudally and secure. See Fig. 29.18
- Centre on: 1–2 cm caudal to the greater tuberosity of the humerus
- Collimate to: (a) midway along the scapula and proximal third of the humerus and (b) approximately 4–5 cm cranial and caudal to the greater tuberosity

If a radiograph of the scapula is required, centre the beam midway between the greater tuberosity and the dorso-caudal aspect of the scapula.

Caudo-cranial

- Animal in trough, in dorsal recumbency
- Extend limb of interest cranially and secure with tie to the table. See Fig. 29.19.
- Centre on: as above
- Collimate to: as above

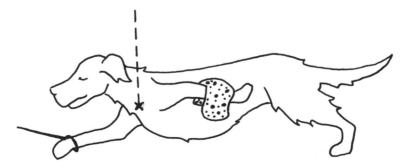

Fig. 29.18   Shoulder lateral view.

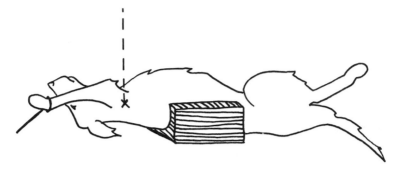

Fig. 29.19 Shoulder caudo-cranial view.

HUMERUS

Lateral

- Position animal the same way as for the lateral shoulder
- Centre on: on the bone, midway between shoulder joint proximally and elbow distally
- Collimate to: include both the shoulder and elbow joint

Caudo-cranial

- Position the animal the same way as for the caudo-cranial shoulder
- Centre on: as above
- Collimate to: as above

ELBOW

Lateral

- Position the animal in the same way as for the shoulder and humerus but ensure the elbow is either in a natural flexed position or fully flexed (e.g. osteochondrosis dessicans)

Some veterinary surgeons prefer the joint to be fully flexed; others favour a more neutral position.
See Fig. 29.20.

- Centre on: middle of medial humeral condyle
- Collimate to: one-third of the way along the humerus proximally and one-third of the way along the radius and ulna distally

RADIOGRAPHY

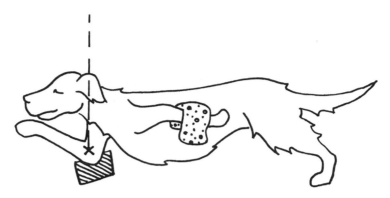

Fig. 29.20   Elbow lateral view.

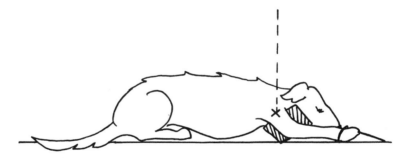

Fig. 29.21   Elbow cranio-caudal view.

Cranio-caudal

- Animal in sternal recumbency
- Draw limb of interest cranially and secure to table with tie
- Place foam pad in between the elbow and the body to prevent rotation. See Fig. 29.21
- Centre on: midline, level with the humeral condyles
- Collimate to: one-third of the way along the humerus proximally and one-third of the way along the radius and ulna distally

RADIUS/ULNA

Lateral and crania-caudal

Both the lateral and cranio-caudal views should be positioned in the same way as the elbow. See Fig. 29.22.

- Centre on: midway between elbow and carpus
- Collimate to: include the elbow and the carpus

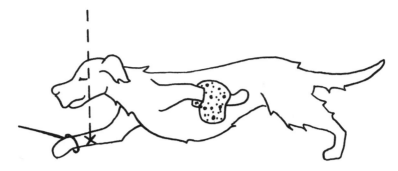

Fig. 29.22   Radius/ulna lateral view.

CARPUS AND FOOT

Lateral and dorso-palmar
These can be positioned in the same way as the elbow and radius/ulna views.

- Centre: over the carpus or middle of foot depending on area of interest
- Collimate: (a) from just proximal to carpus to end of digits
  (b) to include the lateral skin surfaces

If a radiograph of the individual phalanges or pad is required, the toes can be spread apart with tape and a lateral view obtained.

HINDLIMBS

FEMUR

Lateral

- Animal in dorsal recumbency but turned slightly so that the limb of interest falls towards the table
- Place sandbags around the body to maintain the correct position
- Extend the other limb and secure away from limb of interest
- Place small foam wedge under hock to ensure femur is parallel to the cassette. See Fig. 29.23.
- Centre on: midway along femur between stifle and greater trochanter
- Collimate to: include the hip and stifle joints

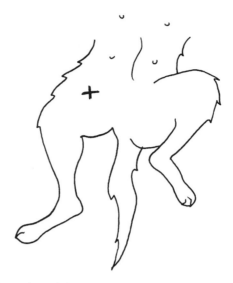

Fig. 29.23 Femur lateral view.

Cranio-caudal

- Animal in trough, in dorsal recumbency
- Extend limb of interest and secure using tie and sandbag
- Secure other limb out of the way. See Fig. 29.24
- Centre on: midway along femur between stifle and greater trochanter
- Collimate to: include the hip and stifle joints

STIFLE

Lateral and cranio-caudal

- Position animal in the same way as for the femur. See Fig. 29.25
- Centre: just distal to the femoral condyles
- Collimate to: include the proximal one-third of the femur and distal one-third of tibia/fibula

TIBIA AND FIBULA

Lateral and cranio-caudal

- Position animal in the same way as for the femur and stifle
- Centre: midway between tarsus and stifle
- Collimate to: include the stifle and hock joints

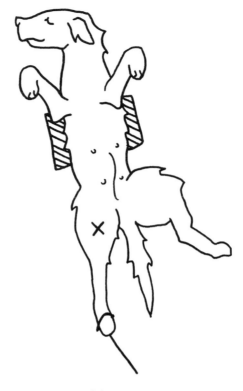

Fig. 29.24 Femur cranio-caudal view.

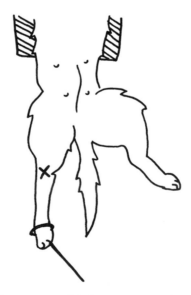

Fig. 29.25 Stifle cranio-caudal view.

RADIOGRAPHY

HOCK AND FOOT

Lateral and dorso-plantar

- Position in the same way as femur, stifle and tibia/fibula
- Centre: over the tarsus or foot depending on the area of interest
- Collimate: (a) just proximal to hock to end of toes (b) lateral skin surfaces

CHAPTER 30

THE PROCESSING OF RADIOGRAPHS

Although many practices now have automatic processors it is still important that nurses are able to manually process films and understand the procedure involved.

Radiographs may be processed by two different methods:

- Manually with tanks (wet processing)
- Automatically using processor machines (dry processing)

The processing procedure consists of five stages:

- Development
- Rinsing (omitted in automatic processing)
- Fixing
- Washing
- Drying

Processing must be carried out in the dark, under safe light conditions because the X-ray film is sensitive to light before it is exposed. Exposure to white light before processing causes the film to turn entirely black.

DEVELOPMENT PROCEDURE

During development, the *exposed* silver bromide crystals in the emulsion are 'reduced' or converted in to grains of *black* metallic silver. When developing a film, always ensure that the following are carried out in this order:

(1) Correct temperature of the solution: 20°C (68°F)
(2) Solution has been agitated (prevents air bubbles and uneven development)
(3) The level of the solution is high enough in the tanks
(4) The film is left in for the correct time (3–5 minutes)

(5) The lid is replaced during development and immediately afterwards – to prevent oxidation of the developer solution

RINSING

Immediately after development, the film must be rinsed in the water tank before being put into the fixer. This removes surplus developing chemicals to prevent contamination of the fixer solution.

The film should be placed in the rinse tank for about 10 seconds.

FIXING

Fixing of the film is required for several reasons:

- The film is still sensitive to white light and must be 'fixed'
- It prevents the film from continuing to be developed
- It removes the unexposed silver bromide crystals
- It hardens the emulsion
- Makes the image permanent

Fixer becomes exhausted (due to the build up of silver bromide ions). Exhaustion happens quicker to fixer than it does to developer.

The speed of fixing increases with high temperatures and with agitation. Fixer temperature is not critical as long as it remains below 21°C. (Above this and temperature staining may occur).

After 10 seconds in the fixer the light may be turned on to view the film. However, total fixing should be at least 10 minutes.

WASHING

After fixing the film, it must be washed for 15–30 minutes. This is to remove residual chemicals that in time would cause fading and yellow/brown staining of the film. Washing is best performed by placing the film in the hanger in a tank of circulating water.

DRYING

Films need to be dried in a *dust free* environment. The film must be removed from its hanger to ensure that the edges dry also.

Films are usually removed from the hanger and then clipped to a line over the sink, taking care that they do *not* touch other films.

Warm air-drying cabinets are available for this purpose. (They are expensive and not widely used.)

PROCESSING NONSCREEN FILMS

Because the emulsion on nonscreen film is thicker, it takes longer for the chemicals to penetrate. This means that non-screen film takes longer to process.

Development time should be increased by about 1 minute and fixing increased by several minutes.

THE MANUAL PROCESSING PROCEDURE

(1) Check the developer and fixer levels
(2) Check the developer and stir
(3) Ensure that hands are clean and dry
(4) Switch on the safe light and load the film hanger with the exposed film
(5) Place the film in the developer, agitate slowly and gently, and replace the lid
(6) Develop for 3–5 minutes
(7) Remove the film from the developer and drain (over the developer tank) to remove excess liquid from the film and hanger
(8) Rinse film immediately before putting into fixer
(9) Place the film in the fixer, after 30 seconds the light may be switched on to check the film. Then fix for a further 10 minutes
(10) Remove the film from the fixer and rinse for 15–30 minutes in running water
(11) Remove the film from the hanger and allow to dry

AUTOMATIC PROCESSORS

Automatic processors only have three tanks: the developer, the fixer and washer dryer.

The films pass through a system of rollers in the machine. The rinsing phase between the developer and fixer is omitted due to the 'squeegee' effect of the rollers. In the wash tank, the water flows at a rate of around 6 l/min so that any contaminants are washed away. The developer and fixer are stored in reservoir tanks and measured quantities are pumped into the appropriate tanks.

Replenishment rate of the chemicals is adjusted to suit film throughput, i.e. the more films that are developed the more replenishing takes place.

PROCEDURE

(1) Ensure the machine is switched on for about 10 minutes prior to use, to warm up (this may be longer in cold weather)
(2) Use an old, clean film to pass through the processor after the warm-up period to ensure the machine is working and remove dried-on chemicals from the rollers
(3) In the darkroom with the safe light on remove the exposed film from the cassette and feed gently into the processor
(4) Load the empty cassette with new film and firmly close it
(5) Ensure all of the film has disappeared into the processor before switching the light on

At the end of the day, the machine should be turned off and the rollers wiped to remove scum.

Automatic processors should be serviced regularly. The rollers and tanks need cleaning regularly. In most automatic processors, the rollers are easily removed for cleaning.

FILM STORAGE

Unexposed film is sensitive to light and must be stored in a light proof 'film-hopper' or the original film box. Film boxes and loaded cassettes must be kept away from the X-ray area and X-ray film should also be kept away from:

• Chemical fumes

RADIOGRAPHY

- Pressure (always keep boxes of film upright)
- Excessive humidity
- High temperatures

FILM IDENTIFICATION

All radiographs need to be labelled permanently with:

- Patient identification
- Date
- Left/right marker
- Any other relevant details, e.g. time after contrast

Labelling can be performed at any of these three stages:

1. During exposure

Using lead letters or *X-rite*™ tape on the outside of the cassette. A left/right marker should also be used at this time.

2. After exposure

In the darkroom using a white-light marker. A small piece of lead in the corner of the cassette protects the film from being exposed to X-ray photons. This corner can then be exposed to white light from behind a piece of paper with the relevant details written on it. (This is not an acceptable method for BVA/KC hip dysplasia radiographs)

3. After processing

Using a chinograph pencil or adhesive label. This is not a good method and not acceptable for legal cases.

LABELLING FILMS FOR BVA/KC HIP AND ELBOW SCORING

Radiographs taken for submission to the BVA/KC must be labelled with:

- The dog's kennel club number
- Date
- Left/right marker

Absolutely no other information is allowed. Acceptable methods of identification for this scheme are only those used at the time of exposure, i.e. lead letters or X-rite tape.

CHAPTER 31

APPRAISAL OF THE FILM

To enable accurate interpretation of the finished film, it is essential that the correct area of the animal has been radiographed *and* that the finished radiographs are of a high diagnostic quality, with good contrast between the body structures and tissues. They must be of clear, sharp quality and have no misleading artefacts.

This requires:

- Correct exposure settings
- Good and standardised processing methods

ASSESSING THE QUALITY OF THE RADIOGRAPH

When the film is developed, the VN should examine it before handing it over to the VS. It is better that the VN admits at the outset if the film has a fault, and suggests that another X-ray is taken than that the VS is given a bad, unreadable, nondiagnostic film.

The radiograph should always be viewed on a viewing box in a dimly lit room. Assessing the radiograph should be done in a step-by-step way.

The following procedure can be used both when checking the films but also when writing up the radiographic case logs:

(1) Positioning: is the part rotated, is it the right area?
(2) Centring: is the primary beam centred on the area of interest?
(3) Collimation: is it 100%, 75%, 50%, 25% or 0%?
(4) Exposure: is it under- or over-exposed?
(5) Processing: is it under- or over-exposed, are there any chemical splashes?
(6) Labelling: is there a left/right marker, date and patient details?

(7) Extraneous marks: are there any white specks, finger-prints, or scratches?

(8) Overall assessment: 'this is a great film of excellent diagnostic quality,' or 'this is a poor film of little diagnostic value, better go and do it again!'

FILM FAULTS – GENERAL RULES

It is important firstly to know the correct methods of setting exposures and processing film and secondly, to recognise film faults and know how to correct them.

Dark films

Remember that overly dark radiographs are over-exposed or over-developed – think of them as being burnt if it helps! This is all very well, but how is it possible to tell if it is over-*exposed* or over-*developed*? The metal left/right marker will reveal the answer. Even if the film is over-exposed, the metal marker should still show up white. If it has been over-developed, even the metal marker will appear darker.

Pale films

What about pale films? Easy, they are under-exposed or under-developed! It is possible to tell the difference here because even on under-exposed films, the exposed areas (around the body) should still be black because even the smallest exposure of X-ray photons on a film will cause blackening. The fault can be identified using the 'finger test'.

- Place a finger between the film and the light viewer in an exposed area that does not contain any part of the animal's body. If it is possible to see the finger through the film, the radiograph is under-developed.

The most common cause of pale films is due to under-development because the processing chemicals are old and exhausted.

Blurred image

The most common cause of blurring of the image is because the animal was moving at the time of exposure. It occurs most commonly because of respiratory movements and sometimes

Table 31.1   Common film faults.

Colour	
Too dark	Over-exposure (reduce kV)
	Over-development
	Developer temperature too high
	Excessive fog
Too pale	Under-exposure
	Developing time too short
	Developing temperature too low
	Developer exhausted
	Developer too dilute

Faulty contrast	
Too high	kV too low
Too low	kV too high
	Under-developed
	Excessive fog
Poor detail	Penumbra effect
	Short FFD
	Object–film distance too great
	Uneven screen film contact
	Patient movement
	Grid lines
	No grid
Fog	Bad storage
	Chemicals
	Radiation
	Light (wrong filter)
Stained films	Insufficient rinsing
Yellow (diachronic fog)	Exhausted fixer

Artefacts	
Streaking	Lack of agitation
	Dirty processing hangers
	Insufficient rinsing
	Drying (watermarks)
Crimp marks (crescent shape)	Mishandling
	(Before exposure – black or white
	Before development – black)
Abrasion marks	Mishandling
	Dirty rollers
Static marks	Black streaks (lightening)
	Bad handling techniques
Developer splashes	Black spots
Fixer splashes	White spots
Screen marks	White (dust specks on screen)
Finger marks	Dark or light fingerprints

due to inadequate restraint of the patient. Try always to keep the time of exposure as short as possible.

The penumbra effect also causes blurring and distortion of the image. This occurs either due to a reduced film-focal distance (FFD) or long object–film distance.

Extraneous marks

Extraneous marks are white specks, scratches, etc. on the finished film. Bad screen handling and maintenance are the most common cause of this. Clean screens regularly and take care when loading and unloading films from the cassette. Table 31.1 identifies some of the common film faults.

RADIOGRAPHY

CHAPTER 32

CONTRAST STUDIES

Contrast studies may be required to gain additional information about structures that are radiolucent or are masked by adjacent or overlying structures. Contrast studies are useful for obtaining information about hollow organs, such as the size, shape and position of them. The VN must be aware of the different types of contrast available, their suitability for particular procedures and the patient preparation and administration of them.

There are two methods of providing contrast:

- Positive contrast
- Negative contrast

POSITIVE CONTRAST RADIOGRAPHY

Positive contrast solutions are *radio-opaque* and so appear *white* on the finished film. They work because they consist of elements of high atomic numbers and absorb a large proportion of the X-ray beam.

Two types of positive contrast preparations available:

- Barium sulphate
- Water soluble iodine-based preparations

BARIUM SULPHATE

This is a white, chalky substance, which is available as liquid, paste or powder. It is used exclusively for gastrointestinal tract studies and it provides excellent mucosal detail. Barium preparations are usually quite tasty and can be administered by mouth; either directly by syringe or stomach tube or mixed in with food. Barium preparations can cause pneumonia if aspirated and should not be used if a perforation along the gastrointestinal system is suspected because they causes adhesions and granulomas.

WATER SOLUBLE IODINE-BASED PREPARATIONS

- Ionic agents
- Nonionic agents

Ionic agents

Ionic iodine-based agents are water soluble and so they may be safely injected into the blood vessels. They may be used in a wide range of situations including:

- Intravenous urography
  - They are excreted rapidly by the kidneys and so are used for intravenous urinary studies (IVU) where they provide excellent outline of the upper urinary tract
- Cystography and urethrography
  - These agents are also frequently used to perform retrograde urethrography or cystography, by injecting the contrast via a urinary catheter into the lower urinary tract
- Angiography
  - Injected intravenously to demonstrate certain areas of the vascular system
- Arthrography
  - Injected into joints to show up abnormalities in joint spaces

Nonionic iodine preparations

Nonionic iodine-based solutions may be used for urinary studies, etc., but they are very much more expensive and are mainly used for myelography. These are required because they do not irritate the spinal cord.

These preparations are classified according to the concentration of iodine in mg/ml. For example Conray 420 contains 420 mg iodine/ml.

NEGATIVE CONTRAST AGENTS

Negative contrast appears *black* on the finished radiograph because it is radiolucent. It consists of gases – room air, oxygen, carbon dioxide or nitrous oxide. Negative contrast studies are useful for showing the position of organs, tumours within organs and urinary calculi. Room air is most frequently used and pneumocystograms would be the most common procedure carried out using this method of contrast.

DOUBLE CONTRAST STUDIES

This contrast study uses both positive and negative contrast agents to create good mucosal detail of organs without obliterating small foreign bodies. A small amount of a positive contrast agent is administered into an organ, lining its internal surface, followed by a larger amount of air.

PATIENT PREPARATION PRIOR TO CONTRAST STUDIES

(1) Withhold food for at least 24 hours – prior to barium studies and intravenous urograms.
(2) Administer enema – prior to colonography, IVU, cystography and urethrography (because faeces will obscure abdominal features).
(3) Obtain plain views of the affected area first – to check any previously overlooked pathology and for comparison with the contrast radiograph.
(4) Warm the contrast medium first if necessary. This is especially important when administering intravenously or for myelography. The required amount can be drawn up into a syringe and then placed in a kidney bowl containing warm water.

CONTRAST RADIOGRAPHY TECHNIQUES

Gastrointestinal tract

- A barium swallow is used to evaluate the oesophagus and/or stomach (gastrogram) by giving the contrast medium by mouth.
- If a megaoesophagus is suspected the liquid barium may be added to tinned meat for the patient to eat (barium meal).
- The stomach may be further evaluated by a positive contrast gastrogram. The barium may be administered by syringe or stomach tube. Better mucosal detail is seen using a double contrast gastrogram. The liquid barium is followed by introduction of room air.

- The small intestine can be assessed by performing a 'barium series', in which radiographs are taken at intervals after the barium administration.
- The large intestine may be studied in the following ways:
  - Negative contrast study using air only (pneumocolon)
  - Positive contrast study using a barium enema
  - Double contrast study using barium and air.

Urogenital tract

- Intravenous urography (IVU) can be used to evaluate the kidneys and ureters. A water-soluble iodine-based contrast agent (e.g. Conray or urografin) is injected intravenously and is rapidly excreted via the kidney. Radiographs are taken in a series to highlight the kidneys and the ureters.
- Contrast cystography can be used to study the bladder by the following three ways:
  - (a) Negative contrast cystography (pneumocystogram) using air injected into the bladder via a urinary catheter
  - (b) Positive contrast cystography using water soluble iodine contrast medium via urinary catheter
  - (c) Double contrast cystography using (a) and (b) in combination.
- The urethra can be studied by retrograde urethrography in male animals and retrograde vagino-urethrography in females. The urinary catheter is inserted into the urethra but pushed no further than the very caudal end of the urethra

The spine

Spinal disease can be investigated by myelography. Contrast medium is injected into the subarachnoid space which surrounds the spinal cord and contains cerebrospinal fluid (CSF). Special water-soluble *nonionic* iodine preparations are used (Iohexol, 'Omnipaque') to minimise irritation. There are two approaches used to inject the contrast – cisternal puncture and lumbar puncture.

Procedure – cisternal puncture

(1) The animal is anaesthetised and plain radiographs of the spine are taken.

(2)   The correct amount of contrast medium is drawn up (0.3 ml/kg).

(3)   An area approximately 8 cm × 8 cm centred over the cisterna magna is clipped and surgically prepared.

(4)   The animal is placed in lateral recumbency with the spine close to the edge of the table and the table tilted slightly to elevate the head.

(5)   The neck is flexed ensuring the nose is parallel to the table. This helps to open up the gap between the skull and the atlas vertebra. The flexing of the neck will cause the endotracheal tube to kink, therefore a reinforced or armoured tube should be used or temporarily remove the tube during this procedure.

(6)   Monitor the animal's respiration to ensure adequate ventilation at all times. The injection of the contrast sometimes causes temporary apnoea.

(7)   The VS will then insert a spinal needle into the subarachnoid space. After withdrawal of the stylet cerebrospinal fluid will drip from the hub of the spinal needle. The contrast agent is then injected slowly. During this procedure it is essential that the head is kept in the same position throughout or the spinal cord may be severed.

(8)   After injection of the contrast medium the needle is removed and the neck is extended. The table may be tilted more to encourage the flow of the contrast medium.

(9)   Radiographs are then taken of the spine.

Procedure – lumbar puncture
If the lesion is more caudal then often a lumbar myelogram is performed.

(1)   The animal is usually placed in sternal recumbency for preparation of the site.

(2)   An area approximately 8 cm × 8 cm is clipped over the 3rd to 5th lumbar vertebrae. Injection is either between L3–4 or L4–5 vertebrae.

(3)   The area is cleaned surgically and the animal positioned laterally with hind legs pulled cranially or in sternal recumbency with the hindlegs again pulled cranially. The positioning helps to open the gap between the vertebrae.

(5)   The veterinary surgeon then places a spinal needle into the subarachnoid space. Often little cerebrospinal fluid is

seen but the animal may 'twitch' its hindlegs, indicating correct position of the needle.

(6) The contrast medium is injected as before and several radiographs are taken.

(7) After myelography it is important that the animal recovers with its head elevated. If a lot of contrast medium is allowed to flow into the brain there is a risk of seizures.

Heart

Angiocardiography under general anaesthesia may help in the diagnosis of some heart and vascular disease.

- Nonselective angiocardiography involves injection of a bolus of contrast via a catheter in the cephalic or jugular vein
- Selective angiography involves the administration of contrast directly into the required heart chamber

Portal venography

Certain liver problems can be diagnosed be portal venography. Under general anaesthesia a laparotomy is performed. An internal vein is catheterised and the contrast injected. Radiographs show the passage of the hepatic portal vein. (Fluoroscopy is most commonly used for this procedure).

Arthrography

This is performed under general anaesthesia. Contrast is injected into the relevant joint via a needle and syringe. Strict asepsis is required when preparing the site so that bacteria are not introduced.

Fistulography

Contrast can be introduced into a sinus tract for their evaluation.

FURTHER READING

Douglas, S.W., Herrtage, M.E., and Williamson, H.D. (1987) *Principles of Veterinary Radiography*, 4th edn. Bailliere Tindall, London.

Lee, R. (ed.) (1995) *BSAVA Manual of Small Animal Diagnostic Imaging*. BSAVA, Gloucestershire, UK.

SECTION 6
LABORATORY TECHNIQUES

CHAPTER 33

INTRODUCTION – THE LABORATORY

The VN should not only be familiar with running samples on modern biochemical and haematological machines but also be able to carry out simple but vital procedures in the laboratory. This section describes these simple procedures for easy reference.

HEALTH AND SAFETY

There are many potential hazards in the laboratory. It is essential that protective and safety clothing is worn when carrying out procedures in the laboratory

- Gloves should always be worn when dealing with samples
- Protective goggles should be worn when using the Bunsen burner
- *Never* eat or drink in the laboratory
- Clinical waste should be disposed of correctly

USING THE MICROSCOPE

(1) Always start with the lowest magnification lens
(2) Ensure the light is turned down low before switching on, this extends the life of the bulb
(3) Place the microscope slide (the correct way up) on the mechanical stage
(4) With binocular microscopes, adjust the eyepieces so that only one image is seen
(5) Increase the light intensity and adjust the condenser for optimal illumination
(6) Move the objective lens down towards the stage, ensuring that the lens does not touch the slide

(7)   Look down the eyepiece(s) and using the coarse and fine focus, adjust the objective lens until the image comes into focus

Now use a higher power objective lens for higher magnification.

When examining smears, immersion oil may be used. Place a drop of oil onto the smear and select the oil immersion lens. Slowly bring the lens down so that it is in the oil. Adjust the focus as necessary. Remember to clean the lens after use.

Vernier scale

The Vernier scale is necessary to relocate an object on the slide. By recording the two measurements, the object can easily be pinpointed again as long as the slide is placed the correct way round on the stage.

Each scale consists of a main scale with millimetre divisions and a smaller Vernier scale reading from 0 to 10.

(1)   The first part of the reading is taken from the main scale. Read the number opposite where the zero on the Vernier scale lies. If it is between two numbers, record the lower number.

(2)   Then look to see which line on the Vernier scale lies directly opposite a line on the main scale. Take the reading off the Vernier scale.

(3)   Repeat for the other scale. The two co-ordinates will be able to exactly locate a point on the slide in much the same way as grid references are used in map reading.

COLLECTION OF SAMPLES

BLOOD

Blood will normally clot after a couple of minutes outside the body. This may be necessary for certain tests where serum instead of plasma is required, otherwise an anticoagulant must be added to prevent coagulation. Table 33.1 compares blood tubes and their uses.

Table 33.1 Comparison of blood tubes and their use.

Anticoagulant	Blood tube colour	Vacutainer colour	Use
EDTA (ethylene diamine tetra-acetic acid)	Pink	Lilac	Haematological examination Optimum concentration = 1 mg/ml
Lithium heparin	Orange	Green	Used for most biochemical estimations, PCV and total plasma protein estimations Clotting is delayed not prevented (sample will clot after 10 hrs)
Fluoride oxalate (sodium fluoride/ potassium oxalate)	Yellow	Grey	Almost solely used for glucose estimation as it helps to prevent glucose metabolism.
Sodium citrate	Purple	Black 1:4 concentration Light blue 1:9 concentration	1:4 concentration = ESR (erythrocyte sedimentation rate) estimation 1:9 concentration = coagulation tests, prothrombin time, etc.
Plain	White	Red	No anticoagulant (for collecting serum)

Notes on collection

- Insufficient anticoagulant will result in the sample clotting. Always ensure the blood tubes are filled accurately.
- Haemolysis (breaking up of red blood cells releasing haemoglobin) can easily occur, which may affect the results:
  - Abnormally low RBC count low PCV (due to the destruction of RBCs).
  - Interfere with the photometric biochemical estimations. This is because of the strong red colour of the plasma.
  - Abnormally high total protein level when measurements are taken using a refractometer.

See Table 33.2 for methods of collection and tests to be performed.

Ensure the animal has been starved for at least 8–12 hours before taking the sample to prevent collection of a lipaemic sample. The lipids in the blood give it a cloudy white appearance, this will also affect the results:

- Causes falsely elevated biochemistry values, because of the effect of the resultant turbidity of the sample on light transmission in photometric measurements

URINE

Notes on collection

- Jam jars or ice cream pots, etc., should not be used for urine collection as these may affect the results
- Ensure sterility at all times especially when collecting a sample for bacteriology

Once a urine sample has been obtained:

- Examine within 1 hour, or
- Refrigerate and examine within 24 hours, or
- Use a preservative and examine within 2 days

A list of preservatives is given in Table 33.3.

Table 33.2 Methods of collection and tests to be performed.

Method	Containers for collection	Tests
Mid-stream free catch	Sterile kidney dish Sterile pot (20 ml sterilin pot)	Dipstick (biochemistry) Sediment
Catheterisation	Sterile kidney dish Sterile pot (20 ml sterilin pot)	Dipstick Sediment Bacteriology
Cystocentesis	Sterile pot (20 ml sterilin pot)	Dipstick Sediment Bacteriology

Table 33.3 Preservatives for urine.

Preservatives		Analysis
Toluene	Enough should be added so that there is a thin film on top of the urine Care – toxic	Biochemistry
Formalin	Add 1 drop of 10% formal saline to 2.5 ml urine Care – toxic	Good for examining urinary sediment, but interferes with biochemical tests Kills bacteria
Thymol	Add 1 mg/ml of urine Will preserve sample up to 24 hours	Biochemistry except glucose estimations Kills bacteria
Boric acid	Sterile universal containers containing boric acid are available The only preservative suitable for culturing bacteria Add 0.5 g/28 ml of urine	Bacteriology and sediment examination Preserves bacteria and prevents multiplication for up to 4 days Also preserves casts and cells

Table 33.4 Methods of collection, preservation and tests to be performed on faeces.

Collection	Preservation	Tests
Must be in screw cap container that is airtight Avoid contamination with other materials such as grass, soil, etc. Completely fill the container to prevent dehydration A rectal sample may be obtained if necessary	Store in the fridge, or add 10% formalin but then the sample can not be used for trypsin or bacteriological tests	Direct faecal smear for undigested fibres Worm egg count Sediment and flotation (ova count)

FAECES

Examination of the faeces must take place as soon as the sample is collected to minimise changes, e.g. eggs hatching, dehydration. Table 33.4 lists methods of collection, preservation and tests to be performed.

LAB TEST PROTOCOLS

There are some tests that are performed by outside laboratories. Each laboratory will have its own requirements on how samples are to be collected and sent. Listed below are common tests performed and collection methods are usually the same for each laboratory. If in doubt, contact the specific laboratory.

ACTIVATED CLOTTING TIME (ACT)

(1) Preheat block and tubes (containing Fullers earth) to 37°C.
(2) Take 2 ml of blood into one of the tubes and mix well.
(3) Place back into the block. Start timing from moment blood sample was taken.
(4) After 1 minute examine sample for clotting and place back in the block.
(5) Then check sample every 10 seconds until blood starts to clot.
(6) Record when the sample first starts to clot.

ADRENOCORTICOTROPHIC HORMONE (ACTH) STIMULATION TEST

A blood sample is taken first (baseline) and then the tetracosactin (Synacthen™) is given intraveneously immediately afterwards. The next sample is taken at least half an hour after the Synacthen™ was given. Synacthen™ should be given by intravenous injection at a dose of half a vial for dogs < 15 kg and 1 vial for dogs > 15 kg. The blood should be centrifuged and the plasma sent to the laboratory.

BILE ACIDS

Bile acids are run routinely in the biochemistry profiles. If a postprandial bile acid sample is needed, check that blood taken was from a fasted patient. If not take a preprandial sample now and then feed the animal (hand or force feed if necessary). A blood sample should then be taken 2 hours after feeding and placed into a heparin tube.

BLOOD CULTURES

Take three samples each an hour apart. Care must be taken to use an aseptic technique, i.e. clip and prepare neck. Raise jugular vein and assess its position by sight, do not touch area with fingers. Take 10 ml of blood. Change needles and inject into blood culture bottle. Label bottle with animal's details including date, time, etc. Store bottles in the fridge prior to submission.

CORTISOL

Serum/plasma sample sent to laboratory.

DIGOXIN LEVELS

Serum.

FELV/FIV

For feline leukaemia virus and feline immunodeficiency virus send either serum or plasma.

FIP

For feline infectious peritonitis serum samples are needed.

HIGH DOSE DEXAMETHASONE SUPPRESSION TEST (HDDST)

Blood samples should be collected into heparin tubes at 0 hours, 3 hours and 8 hours postinjection. Dexamethasone should be injected at a dose of 0.1 mg/kg by intravenous injection.

Note: A soluble dexamethasone preparation such as Dexadreson™ (2 mg/ml) should be used.

LOW DOSE DEXAMETHASONE SCREENING TEST (LDDST)

Blood samples need to be collected into heparin tubes at 0 hours, 3 hours and 8 hours postinjection. Dexamethasone should be injected intravenously at a dose of 0.01 mg/kg. The blood samples should be centrifuged and the plasma sent to the laboratory.

Note: A soluble dexamethasone preparation such as Dexadreson™ (2 mg/ml) should be used.

TAURINE LEVELS

Laboratories can run taurine along with 15 other amino acids using a chromatography method on serum.

TOTAL T4 (THYROXINE)

Test is run on serum/plasma samples sent to laboratory.

THYROID HORMONE STIMULATION TEST

Take blood samples into heparin tubes at 0 hours and 6 hours postinjection. Thyroid stimulating hormone (TSH) should be given by intravenous injection at a dose of 0.1 unit/kg (TSH contains 2 units/ml), up to a maximum dose of 5 units or 2.5 ml.

VON WILLEBRAND'S DISEASE

Blood should be put into a citrate tube for the laboratory.

CHAPTER 34

BLOOD TESTS

BLOOD TESTS REQUIRING LITTLE EQUIPMENT

HAEMATOCRIT OR PACKED CELL VOLUME (PCV)

Used to find the percentage of the blood that is occupied by red blood cells (RBCs). It is used to assess anaemia or dehydration.

BLOOD SMEAR

Performed so that the individual cells may be examined.

STAINING BLOOD SMEARS

Enables white blood cells to be seen more easily.

DIFFERENTIAL WHITE CELL COUNT

Examination of the blood smear and calculation of the different types of white blood cell present

TOTAL CELL COUNTS

Calculation of the number of red and white blood cells. A counting chamber (haemocytometer) is used.

METHOD FOR MEASURING PACKED CELL VOLUME (PCV)

Equipment:

- Microhaematocrit tubes (red mark = coated with heparin, blue mark = plain)
- Blood in EDTA tube
- 'Cristaseal'

- Centrifuge
- Hawksley Microhaematocrit Reader
- Tissues and disposable gloves

Method:

Put on gloves
   (1) Invert the blood tube to ensure the contents have mixed thoroughly
   (2) Fill two capillary tubes three-quarters full with blood (leave 10–15 mm unfilled)
   (3) Wipe the outside and then seal the end of the tubes with 'Cristaseal™'
   (4) Place the two tubes opposite each other in order to balance the centrifuge (ensure open end points inwards!) and secure the safety plate
   (5) Centrifuge for 5 minutes at 10 000 rev/min
   (6) Place tube on Hawksley™ Microhaematocrit Reader
   (7) Place bottom of RBC column on baseline of scale
   (8) Move the tube until the top of the plasma is level with the upper sloping line
   (9) Adjust the movable line so that it is at the top of the RBC column
   (10) Read off the percentage value on the scale

The percentage may also be read by measuring the length of the red blood cells and dividing it by the total length of the plasma, buffy coat and red cells. Multiply this by 100 to get the percentage.

PREPARATION OF A BLOOD SMEAR

Equipment:

- Microscope slides
- 'Spreader'
- Blood (in EDTA)
- Alcohol
- Capillary tube
- Disposable gloves and tissues

Method:

Put on gloves
   (1) Clean the slide with alcohol to degrease it: ensure that it is dry

(2) Place slide on pale background
(3) Place small drop of well-mixed blood on one end of the slide using a capillary tube
(4) Place spreader just in front of the blood at an angle of 45°
(5) Move spreader back into the blood until the blood spreads along the edge of the spreader
(6) Then move the spreader forward in a single, smooth, rapid motion
(7) Air-dry the smear
(8) Either stain when dry or fix in absolute methanol for 5 minutes, then staining can be postponed for up to 3 days

Figure 34.1 shows the method of making a blood smear.

It should be possible to assess the smear and diagnose any faults using Table 34.1.

STAINING BLOOD SMEARS

The most commonly used stains are from the Romanowsky group.

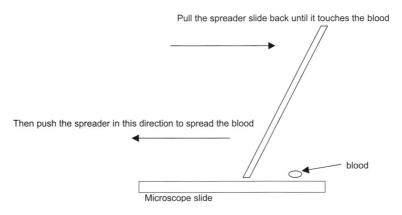

Pull the spreader slide back until it touches the blood

Then push the spreader in this direction to spread the blood

blood

Microscope slide

Fig. 34.1 Making a blood smear.

Table 34.1 Problems with blood smears.

Faults	Cause
Smear too long	Too much blood, blood is anaemic, spreader angle too small
Smear too short	Too little blood, spreader angle too great
Alternate thick/thin bands	Uneven spreader edge/jerky motion when spreading
Areas of no blood, patchy	Grease on slide
Smear thick and narrow	Blood has not had time to spread along spreader

LEISHMAN'S STAINING METHOD

Equipment:

- Dish
- Rack
- Leishman's stain
- Distilled water

Method:

(1) Place slide on rack, smear uppermost.
(2) Cover with Leishman's stain. Leave 1–2 minutes to fix smear.
(3) Cover slide with *twice* volume of buffered distilled water (pH 6.8).
(4) Gently rock slide from side to side to evenly mix solution. Leave for 10–15 minutes.
(5) Wash off slide with the buffered distilled water. Flood slide for 1 minute until pinkish tinge just appears.
(6) Pour off the water and stand the slide upright on blotting paper to dry.

GIEMSA STAIN

Useful for identifying particular cells or parasites (*Haemobartonella felis*).

(1) Dip the slide in methanol for a few seconds to fix the cells.
(2) Flood the slide with Giemsa and leave for 30 minutes.
(3) Rinse the slide with distilled water and leave upright to dry.

DIFF-QUIK™ STAIN

A very quick and easy method of staining smears although not as good as Leishman's.

Three solutions are required:

- Solution A – fixative (methanol) light blue
- Solution B – stain (eosin) red
- Solution C – stain (thiazine dye) purple
  (1) Dip slide into solution A five times.
  (2) Remove and dip into solution B five times.

(3) Remove and dip into solution C seven times (helps to stain the platelets if left longer).

(4) Rinse the slide with distilled water and leave upright to air dry.

DIFFERENTIAL WHITE CELL COUNT

Equipment:

- Stained blood smear
- Immersion oil
- Microscope
- Chart to count cells

Method:

(1) Prepare a fresh blood smear and stain with Leishman's or Diff-Quick™.

(2) Apply a small drop of immersion oil to the edge of the smear.

(3) Move along the edge of the smear using the 'battlement' method.

(4) Count and record the different types of leucocyte.

(5) Count at least 100 cells for every 10 000 cells in the total white cell count. (The more cells that are counted the more accurate the result will be.)

(6) Then work out the percentage for each type of cell found.

Table 34.2 shows normal ranges for white blood cell differential tests.

TOTAL CELL COUNTS

Equipment:

- Improved Neubauer haemocytometer with cover slip

Table 34.2 Normal ranges for white blood cell differential test.

White blood cell (WBC)	Dog (%)	Cat (%)
Neutrophils		
• adult	70	60
• immature	0.8	0.5
Eosinophils	4	5
Basophils	1	1
Lymphocytes	20	32
Monocytes	5	3

- Thoma pipettes (special pipettes to allow correct dilution of blood)
- Diluents for white cell and red cell count
- Blood in preserved in EDTA
- Disposable gloves and tissues

Preparing the haemocytometer:

(1) Ensure the haemocytometer is dry.
(2) Place the cover slip over the counting square in the centre of the haemocytometer.
(3) Press firmly on the edges of the cover slip and move back and forward to squeeze the air out between the cover slip and haemocytometer. This may be easier if the two surfaces are slightly damp.
(4) Once 'Newtons rings' appear the cover slip will be stuck to the haemocytometer.
(5) This ensures the space between the counting chamber on the haemocytometer and the cover slip is exactly 1 mm, thus ensuring that the calculation is correct.

RED BLOOD CELL COUNT

Diluent must be isotonic to prevent haemolysis. Table 34.3 shows different types of diluents.

Thoma pipette (RBC) method
The Thoma pipette with the red bead must be used to ensure accurate dilution.

(1) Put on gloves.
(2) Mix blood gently by inverting several times.
(3) Draw up blood to 0.5 mark using the tubing and 1 ml syringe (do not mouth pipette).
(4) Wipe outside of pipette.
(5) Draw up diluent to 101 mark, wipe outside.

Table 34.3 Different types of diluents.

Diluent	Notes
0.9% saline	Perform count soon after dilution
Hayem's solution	Can cause agglutination of cells ('clumping' together)
Dacie's formol-citrate solution	Helps to preserve sample from agglutination for up to 1 hour

(6) Mix gently by rotating the pipette.

(7) Discard diluent in stem by wiping the end gently on a tissue.

(8) Fill counting chamber by gently touching the tip to the small gap between the counting chamber and the cover slip.

(9) Place chamber under microscope.

(10) Allow cells to settle for 2–3 minutes.

(11) Examine under high power and low illumination.

Or

Add 0.02 ml of blood to 4 ml diluent using ordinary graduated pipette

Calculation of RBC

Multiply the number of cells counted in five large squares marked with 'R' (see Fig. 34.2) by 10 000. This will indicate the number of cells per cubic millimetre.

WHITE BLOOD CELL COUNT

Diluent

The diluent for white blood cells is 1 ml of 1% gentian violet (stains the cells) mixed with 2 ml of 2% glacial acetic acid made up to 100 ml by the addition of 97 ml saline or distilled water. This will destroy the red blood cells, thereby making it easier to count the white cells.

Thoma pipette (WBC) method:

Use the Thoma pipette with the white bead to ensure accurate dilution.

(1) Put on gloves.

(2) Mix blood gently by inverting several times.

(3) Draw up blood to 0.5 mark using the tubing and 1 ml syringe (do not mouth pipette).

(4) Wipe outside of pipette.

(5) Draw up diluent to 11 mark, wipe the outside.

(6) Mix by gently rotating the pipette.

(7) Leave for 10 minutess to allow haemolysis and staining to occur.

(8) Discard diluent in the stem by wiping the tip gently on a tissue.

(9) Fill counting chamber as before.

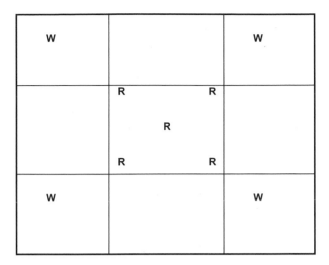

Fig. 34.2   The haemocytometer grid.

(10) Place chamber under the microscope.
(11) Allow the cells to settle for 2–3 minutes.
(12) Examine under high power and low illumination.

Calculation of WBC
Multiply the number of cells in the four outer squares marked with 'W' (see Fig. 34.2) by 50. This will give the number of WBC per cubic millimetre.

White blood cell count using the Unopette™ method

(1)   Fill the Unopette™ pipette with blood – 25 µl.
(2)   Place the pipette into the reservoir of diluent.
(3)   Invert the reservoir to rinse the pipette and to mix the solution thoroughly.
(4)   Allow to stand for 10 minutes to allow haemolysis of the red blood cells.
(5)   Discard the first few drops then fill the chamber as before.
(6)   Examine under high power.

Unopettes™ are also available for red cell counts.

CHAPTER 35

URINE TESTS

Various simple tests can be performed on urine with minimal equipment.

- Dipstick analysis: (biochemical estimations of glucose, protein, ketones, bilirubin and pH, etc.)
- Specific gravity: 'an index of the concentration of substances dissolved in it'
- Examination of the sediment

URINE DIPSTICK TESTS

BM TEST 8 MULTISTIX

This is an eight patch test strip for the determination of nitrite, pH, protein, glucose, ketone bodies, urobilinogen, bilirubin and blood in urine.

Equipment:

- Urine sample
- Multistix (check 'in date')
- Pipette or syringe (1 or 2 ml)
- Disposable gloves and tissue

Method:

(1) Put on disposable gloves.
(2) Take a fresh urine sample (< 4 hours old) and mix thoroughly.
(3) Draw some urine into a pipette or syringe.
(4) Remove one stick and replace lid immediately
(5) Cover each of the patches with urine.
(6) After 60 seconds, compare reaction colours with the colour scale on the label.

If the urine is removed from the sample rather than dipping the stick into it the sample can then be used for other tests.

BM DIABUR TEST 5000

This strip test is used to detect glucose in urine. Levels up to 5000 mg/100 ml (5%) can be detected.
Method:

(1)   Collect urine in a clean container.
(2)   Dip stick briefly and remove excess.
(3)   Read after 2 minutes by comparing test areas with colour scale on the label.

Note: Alternatively the test strip may be wetted by holding directly in the urine stream.
Reading results:
For concentrations less than 1% (i.e. 1000 mg/100 ml), the upper yellow–green scale permits more accurate readings. For higher readings read against the lower light blue row of colours.

SPECIFIC GRAVITY

Specific gravity = weight of a certain volume of a liquid ÷ weight of the same volume of water

Therefore the specific gravity of pure water is 1.000. The specific gravity of urine is an estimation of the concentration ability of the kidney.

MEASURING SPECIFIC GRAVITY USING A REFRACTOMETER

Equipment:

• Urine sample
• Refractometer
• Distilled water
• Tissues
• Disposable gloves
• Pipette or 1 ml syringe

Method:

(1)   Put on disposable gloves.
(2)   Test with distilled water by placing 1–2 drops on the face of the prism and replace the cover.

(3) Look through the eye piece, pointing the refractometer towards the light. Focus scale by rotating rim of eyepiece. The line should cross at the 1.000 mark, if not alter using the scale adjusting screw.

(4) Wipe away water with a piece of soft tissue.

(5) Then repeat procedure using 1–2 drops of urine.

(6) Record result.

(7) Clean refractometer using distilled water.

Note: The refractometer is calibrated for use at room temperature. So urine that has been stored in the fridge should be allowed to come to room temperature before testing. If the urine is particularly concentrated it may give a result which is off the scale. In this case, dilute with same volume of water and take another reading. Double the result to get the actual reading.

Normal range:

- Dog: 1.015–1.045
- Cat: 1.020–1.040

EXAMINATION OF THE URINARY SEDIMENT

The urine sample may be centrifuged so that any solid particles are concentrated into sediment. A normal sample will not usually produce much sediment.

Staining the preparation:

- Leishman's will stain cells
- Gram's stain will stain bacteria
- Sedistain stains all of the sediment

PREPARATION OF THE SEDIMENT

Equipment:

- Fresh urine sample
- Centrifuge and centrifuge tubes
- Sedistain™
- Pipette or 1 ml syringe
- Microscope slide and cover slip
- Disposable gloves

Method:

(1) Centrifuge sample for 5 minutes at 2000 rev/min in a centrifuge tube.
(2) Remove the supernatant fluid leaving a few drops in which to resuspend the sample. ('Flick' the tube to do this).
(3) A drop of Sedistain™ may be added in which to resuspend the sediment and to stain the debris.
(4) Place a few drops on a microscope slide and apply a cover slip (avoiding air bubbles).
(5) Examine under low power and low illumination.

TO PRODUCE A SMEAR OF THE SEDIMENT

Equipment:

- Fresh urine sample that has been centrifuged
- Sedistain™
- Pipette or 1 ml syringe
- Microscope slide and 'spreader'
- Disposable gloves

Method:

(1) Prepare the sample as before.
(2) Place a small drop of the sediment on the slide and smear using the same method as for blood.
(3) Alternatively, use a bacteriological loop to spread the drop evenly over the slide.
(4) Allow the smear to air-dry.
(5) Sedistain™ stain may be used.

The sample may then be examined for crystals, casts, bacteria, cells and blood cells.

CHAPTER 36

FAECAL TESTS

Examination of the faeces must take place as soon as the sample is collected to minimise changes, e.g. eggs hatching, dehydration.

TESTS

- Direct faecal smear for undigested fibres
- Concentration methods for detecting endoparasitic ova
- Worm egg count – McMaster technique

OTHER TESTS

- Ovassay kit – 2 g faeces plus solution to check for ova
- Okokit – tests for occult blood
- Haemastix – tests for blood

PREPARATION OF A DIRECT FAECAL SMEAR

Equipment:

- Fresh faecal sample
- Water or saline
- Microscope slide and cover slip
- Spatula
- Disposable gloves

Method:

Put on gloves.
(1) Place a few drops of water or saline on the microscope slide.
(2) Mix in a small amount of faeces (remove large pieces of debris).

(3) Apply a cover slip (avoiding air bubbles) and examine under low power.

(4) Examine the smear systematically, e.g. from left to right across the smear then move down one field of vision, then examine from right to left and so on.

TESTS FOR IMPAIRED DIGESTION

Various stains may be added to the faecal smear to test for digestion insufficiency. Table 36.1 shows which stains test for various undigested food substances.

CONCENTRATION METHODS FOR DETECTING ENDOPARASITIC OVA

SEDIMENTATION

This method is useful as any ova present will be concentrated into the sediment.

Equipment:

- Fresh faecal sample
- Glass container or jar
- Spatula
- Sieve
- Centrifuge and centrifuge tubes
- Disposable gloves and tissues

Table 36.1   Stains used for various undigested food substances.

Food substance	Stain
Undigested muscle fibres Undigested muscle fibres stain pink and have ragged or broken ends with striations of skeletal muscle and nuclei present. Their presence may indicate deficiency of trypsin. Digested muscle fibres have rounded ends and the striations and nuclei will be faint or absent (cooked muscle fibres also have this appearance, however).	1 drop of 2% eosin solution
Undigested fat globules Undigested fat globules or droplets stain orange-red and may indicate deficiency of lipase.	1 drop of Sudan III solution
Undigested starch granules Undigested starch granules stain blue-black and may appear as flowers or snow flakes. These may indicate deficiency of amylase, but may also be seen in an animal fed on a high biscuit diet.	1 drop of Lugol's iodine solution

Method:

Put on gloves.
(1)   Add 2 g faeces to 30 ml water in a small jar or bottle.
(2)   Mix thoroughly to break up the faecal matter. (Glass beads may be added and the solution shaken vigorously to break up faecal matter.)
(3)   Strain into a conical centrifuge tube to remove gross debris.
(4)   Centrifuge for 3 minutes at 1–1500 rev/min.
(5)   Discard the supernatant fluid and pipette a few drops of the sediment onto a microscope slide. Apply a cover slip avoiding air bubbles.
(6)   Examine under low power.

SEDIMENTATION AND FLOTATION

Use technique above but use a flotation solution instead. After discarding the supernatant fluid, fill the tube completely with a flotation solution. Place a cover slip on top of the meniscus formed and leave for 10 minutes. The eggs will float up to the surface. Thereafter the cover slip can then be transferred directly to the microscope slide.
   Flotation solutions:

• Saturated sugar solution
• Saturated salt solution
• Sodium nitrate solution
• Zinc sulphate

McMASTER TECHNIQUE FOR COUNTING WORM EGGS

This is a quantitative method for determining the number of eggs per gram of faeces. It is not routinely used as any evidence of ova will be treated with appropriate anthelmintics.
   Equipment:

• McMaster counting chamber
• Fresh faecal sample
• Flotation solution
• Pipette or syringe
• Disposable gloves and tissues

Method:

Put on gloves.
(1) Mix 2 g of faeces with 30 ml of a flotation solution.
(2) Place in a screw-top jar (with glass balls).
(3) Shake well for 1–2 minutes.
(4) Strain, stir and pipette solution into both counting chambers.
(5) Examine under low power and count eggs in both chambers.

CALCULATION

X = number of eggs in both chambers.

$X/2 \times 100$ = number of eggs per gram of faeces

CHAPTER 37

BACTERIOLOGY TESTS

TESTS

- Bacterial smear
- Staining of bacterial smears
- Culturing bacteria
- Sensitivity tests

MAKING A BACTERIAL SMEAR

Equipment:

- Microscope slide
- Bunsen burner
- Tongs for holding the slide when heat fixing
- Inoculating loop
- Chinagraph pencil for labelling the slide
- Disposable gloves, face mask, goggles

Method:

(1) Take a clean microscope slide and sterilise it by passing it through a Bunsen burner flame
(2) Allow the slide to cool then apply sample material to the slide
(3) Allow the smear to dry in air
(4) When the smear is dry, fix it by passing it through the flame to kill the bacteria and adhere them to the slide
(5) Before staining use the chinagraph pencil to label the slide and to outline the smear

Table 37.1 outlines the methods for preparing bacterial smears from different types of sample.

Table 37.1 Procedures for making bacterial smears.

Sample characteristics	Procedure
Fluid	Sterilise the inoculating loop in the flame. Then pick up a loop full of fluid and spread it on the slide. Resterilise the loop.
Materials of thicker consistency (e.g. pus or bacterial colony taken from a culture plate)	Place a drop of distilled water on the slide and apply some of the sample with a sterile inoculating loop. Mix the water to produce an emulsion, which can be spread over the slide.
Swab	Spread over the surface of the slide and add a drop of water if it is too dry.

STAINING BACTERIAL SMEARS

The bacterial smear can then be stained to identify different shapes or families of bacteria.

1. METHYLENE BLUE STAINING

This is a simple stain to show the shape of the bacteria.
  Equipment:

- Heat fixed smear
- Methylene blue 1% solution
- Distilled water
- Staining rack
- Disposable gloves

Method:

(1) Put on gloves
(2) Place slide on the rack with smear uppermost
(3) Flood slide with 1% aqueous methylene blue
(4) Leave for 2 minutes
(5) Wash off with distilled water
(6) Leave slide upright to dry

2. GRAM STAIN

Stains Gram-negative and Gram-positive bacteria different colours.

(1) First stage: the *violet* (primary or basic stain) stain stains both types of bacteria.
(2) Second stage: the *mordant* (iodine) fixes the violet stain.

LABORATORY TECHNIQUES

(3) Third stage: the *decoloriser* (alcohol) causes the Gram-negative bacteria to lose their violet colour.

(4) Fourth stage: the *red* stain (carbol fuchsin) stains the Gram-negative organisms red. The Gram-positive organisms remain violet.

Equipment:

• Heat fixed bacterial smear
• Solutions needed: crystal violet
  • Gram's or Lugol's iodine
  • Acetone or industrial methylated spirit
  • Dilute carbol fuchsin (1/10 with distilled water) or safranin 0.5%
• Staining rack
• Distilled water
• Disposable gloves

Method:

(1) Put on gloves
(2) Place the slide on the rack with the smear uppermost
(3) Flood slide with crystal violet solution
(4) Leave 30–60 seconds
(5) Gently rinse the slide with distilled water
(6) Flood with Gram's or Lugol's iodine
(7) Leave 30–60 seconds
(8) Pour off excess iodine and rinse with distilled water
(9) Flood slide with acetone and immediately rinse off with distilled water
(10) Counterstain with dilute carbol fuchsin for 1 minute
(11) Pour off excess stain and rinse with distilled water
(12) Leave slide upright to air dry

Lugol's iodine is more concentrated than Gram's iodine (1 ml Lugol's added to 100 ml water = Gram's iodine). It is used for a darker colour, there is less chance of excessive decolorisation.

3. ZIEHL-NEELSON ACID-FAST STAIN

Used to detect 'acid-fast' organisms, e.g. *Mycobacterium tuberculosis*. They are stained with carbol fuchsin and heated. They are resistant to decolorisation with the acid alcohol and so retain the red colour when counterstained with methylene blue.

Acid-fast bacteria appear bright red on a blue background. Other organisms stain blue.

Ziehl-Neelson's staining technique
Equipment:

- Heat fixed smear
- Bunsen burner
- Staining rack
- Forceps or tongs to hold the slide
- Ziehl-Neelson's carbol fuchsin stain
- Acid alcohol
- Loefflers methylene blue
- Distilled water
- Disposable gloves and goggles

Method:

(1) Hold slide containing smear in a pair of forceps
(2) Cover smear with Ziehl-Neelson's carbol fuchsin
(3) Heat over a Bunsen burner until stain starts to steam (do not let it boil)
(4) Then put slide onto staining rack. Leave for 3–4 minutes then reheat again
(5) After 5–7 minutes from first heating wash stain off under tap
(6) Then apply an acid alcohol
(7) Wash with distilled water (gently) until as much of the red stain as possible has been removed
(8) Cover with the second stain, Loefflers methylene blue
(9) Leave for 1 minute
(10) Then wash off with distilled water
(11) Leave smear to air dry.

Firstly all bacteria stain red. Then acid-alcohol washes red stain off nonacid-fast bacteria. These bacteria then stain red-blue.

CULTURING BACTERIA

Most bacteria can be grown on agar plates at 37°C. The bacteria are spread out over the plate using the streaking out method. This allows single colony identification.

INOCULATING AGAR CULTURE PLATES ('STREAKING OUT' METHOD)

Equipment:

- Agar plate (Petri-dish (sterile) with appropriate agar medium)
- Inoculating loop (Nichrome)
- Bunsen burner
- Bacterial sample
- Disposable gloves, face mask and goggles

Method:

(1) Put on gloves, mask and goggles.

(2) Sterilise the inoculating loop in the Bunsen burner flame until it glows orange.

(3) Pick up the half of the Petri dish containing the media and turn to face upwards.

(4) Smear the sample from the loop or swab over a small area to produce a 'well' of bacteria (well inoculum).

(5) Resterilise the loop in the flame or replace the swab in its container.

(6) With the sterile loop make three to four short strokes all in the same direction away from the well (this will be A). Take care not to tear at or cut the agar.

(6) Resterilise the loop.

(7) Continue in the same way to produce streaks B, C and D. Resterilise the loop between each group of streaks and then again at the end. In this way the bacteria are thinned out, so that by groups C and D, individual colonies of bacteria will grow.

(8) Place the two halves of the Petri dish together, the one containing the medium uppermost.

(9) Label with case details and incubate at 37°C for 18–24 hours. Plates must be laid in the incubator medium side uppermost to prevent condensation contaminating the sample.

Figure 37.1 shows an inoculating plate.

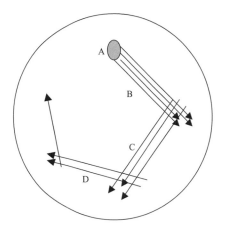

Fig. 37.1 Inoculating plate.

IDENTIFICATION OF BACTERIAL GROWTH MAY DEPEND ON COLONY CHARACTERISTICS

- Any zone of haemolysis in the blood agar around the colony (haemolytic or nonhaemolytic)
- The size of the colony (measurement in mm)
- The colour of the colony (grey, cream, yellow, white, etc.)
- If opaque or translucent
- The shape and consistency (irregular, circular, raised, flat, convex, mucoid, flaky, hard or crusty)
- The odour (sweet, musty, pungent, etc.)

INOCULATING CULTURE PLATES FOR USE WITH SENSITIVITY DISCS

Equipment:
Diagnostic sensitivity testing agar.

Method 1:

(1) Make an inoculum well.
(2) Make strokes from well in three directions across plate to spread sample as evenly as possible without sterilising the loop in between (sterilise only at the beginning and end).

Method 2:

(1) Take a sterile syringe case and add 1 ml of sterile water.

(2) Sterilise the loop and pick up the sample on the loop.

(3) Mix the loop full of sample in sterile water.

(4) Pour over the medium, then rock the dish to spread the sample evenly over the surface. After this pour off the remaining water.

(5) After inoculating the media, the sensitivity discs can then be applied to the surface of the agar using a sterile pair of forceps or a purpose-designed disc dispenser. The plates are then incubated in the normal way.

Sensitivity discs are paper discs impregnated with different antibacterial and antibiotic agents. The discs should be firmly pressed onto the agar surface using sterile forceps (sterilise by passing them through the Bunsen flame). This allows the antibacterial substance to diffuse into the surrounding agar. The plates are incubated at 37°C. Check after 18–24 hours. The agar surface should be covered with bacterial growth except for around discs that contain an antibiotic or antibacterial agent that those bacteria are sensitive to.

It is not completely accurate to record sensitivity in this way because some bacterial substances diffuse out into the media more quickly than others and the concentration of drugs on the discs may not compare to the normal doses given to the patient.

CHAPTER 38

DERMATOLOGY

HOW TO FIND ECTOPARASITES

COLLECTION OF SAMPLES

Many parasitological skin diseases appear clinically very similar to each other and so sampling methods must be undertaken and laboratory analysis carried out for accurate diagnosis.

The veterinary nurse must be confident in obtaining samples and performing the various laboratory tests to aid diagnosis. Good sample quality is essential to get reliable results.

Remember to take appropriate hygiene precautions, i.e. wear gloves, and an apron if necessary. The sample being taken may be zoonotic (e.g. *Sarcoptes*, *Cheyletiella*, ringworm).

The following methods may be performed to collect ectoparasite samples:

- Skin scrapings
- Coat brushings
- Hair plucks
- Tape strips
- Pustular smears
- Ear wax swab

METHODS

Skin scrapings
Skin scrapes are useful to detect the burrowing mites *Sarcoptes scabei* and *Demodex canis*.

(1) Chose a suitable area (usually the edge of the affected area or lesion is better because the mites travel outwards from the centre).
(2) Gently clip hair around the area to be scraped.

(3) Apply a drop of liquid paraffin to the skin surface and a no. 10 scalpel blade.

(4) Squeeze the skin between the fingers so that the area is stable. (This also helps to squeeze the parasites closer to the surface.)

(5) Gently scrape the top layers of the skin surface until pin-pricks of blood are seen oozing from the area. It is important to scrape until blood appears to ensure that the scrape is deep enough.

(6) Transfer the scraped material onto a microscope slide and smear it out so that the sample is not too thick; this will make it easier to see the parasites.

(7) Place a cover slip over the top and examine under low power.

(8) Scan slide methodically until the parasite is found.

(9) Increase magnification as necessary.

(10) Record the Vernier scale readings of any mites found so that they can be relocated if necessary.

Some people prefer to place a few drops of 10% potassium hydroxide (KOH) on to the slide instead of liquid paraffin because it removes (clears) the keratin. However, liquid paraffin is useful because the parasites remain alive, making location of them far easier. Take several scrapings from several sites, using a new blade for each site.

Coat brushings

Coat brushings may reveal fleas and/or their faeces, lice, *Cheyletiella* mites and eggs.

(1) Stand the patient onto a large sheet of white paper

(2) Vigorously brush the coat with the fingers or brush

(3) Collect the dislodged material and transfer some of it onto a microscope slide with some liquid paraffin

(4) Apply a cover slip

(5) Examine under the microscope in the same way as a skin scrape

WET PAPER TEST

Wet a small wad of cotton wool and squeeze all of the excess moisture out of it. Dab this over the remaining sample that is left on the white paper. Flea faeces may be confirmed by the blood-tinged marks on the cotton wool or paper.

HAIR PLUCKS

Hair plucks may be taken and submitted for fungal culture or examined for louse and *Cheyletiella* eggs, which are attached to the hair shaft.

(1) Pluck small amounts of hair from the affected area
(2) Place onto microscope slide with some liquid paraffin if examining for eggs
(3) Place cover slip and examine under low power

When examining hair pluck for the presence of fungal spores (for evidence of ringworm), place sample onto a microscope slide but do not add any liquid paraffin or KOH. Place a cover slip and examine for spores under ×100 or ×400 magnification. It is also possible to examine these hairs under ultraviolet light (Wood's lamp) for fluorescence to confirm *Microsporum canis*

TAPE STRIPS

Clear adhesive tape (e.g. *Sellotape*™) may be used to collect fleas, lice and harvest mites and to demonstrate the presence of microbes such as *Malassezia*.

(1) Choose the area to be tested and if necessary, separate the hairs to allow access to the skin below
(2) Press a length of clear adhesive tape firmly onto the area
(3) Repeat this and then transfer the tape, sticky side down onto a microscope slide for examination under low power
(4) If examining for *Malassezia*, loop the section of tape with the sample on and stick the remaining tape to a microscope slide
(5) Dip the sample into a stain such as Diff-Quick™ or methylene blue and examine under oil immersion for presence of yeasts and fungal hyphae
(6) Unstick the tape and reposition so that the sample is over the slide
(7) Examine under high magnification

PUSTULAR SMEARS

Pustular smears are useful to detect pustular demodectic mange and identification of bacteria from skin lesions.

(1) Squeeze a pustule and transfer the contents directly onto a microscope slide (wear clean gloves to hold skin for bacterial examination)

(3) Smear the contents evenly over the slide with a mounted needle or similar

(4) Apply cover slip and examine under the microscope

EAR WAX

Ear wax can be collected and examined for presence of *Otodectes cyanotis*.

(1) Using a cotton bud, gently collect some of the ear wax from the external ear canal

(2) Transfer the wax onto a microscope slide

(3) Mix the wax with 2–3 drops of liquid paraffin or KOH and break up the clumps using a sterile needle so that the sample is not too thick

(4) Apply cover slip and examine under microscope

EXAMINATION FOR RINGWORM

As previously mentioned, dry plucked hairs can be examined microscopically.

Look for obviously thickened hair shafts under low power and then increase magnification to ×100 or ×400 magnification to visualise fungal spores. A drop of lactophenol cotton blue stain or 'Quink' ink may be added to the sample to make visualisation of the spores easier.

ULTRAVIOLET (WOOD'S LAMP) EXAMINATION

A Wood's lamp uses an ultraviolet light to help detect certain strains of ringworm (50% of *Microsporum canis* show up this way). The dermatophytes fluoresce an apple-green colour when examined under the light.

(1) Switch on the Wood's lamp 5–10 minutes prior to examination to allow it to warm up
(2) Examination should be carried out in a darkened room
(3) Examination with a Wood's lamp can be done either by passing the lamp directly over the coat of the animal or by shining over plucked hairs for at least 3–5 minutes

Remember that a negative Wood's light examination does not rule out ringworm because only a small percentage of ringworm are responsive to UV light and that other rare dermatophytes and certain bacterial infections can also fluoresce.

FUNGAL CULTURES

Hair pluckings can be collected and carefully inoculated using sterile forceps onto one of two media: Sabouraud's agar or Dermatophyte Test Medium (DTM is available in commercial fungal culture kits for use in practices, with the name Dermafyt™). The unit containing the culture should be sealed with biohazard tape and kept at room temperature for 7–10 days. It should be checked daily for the appearance of a white colony and a red coloration of the medium, which indicates the presence of a dermatophyte. If there is no growth after 3 weeks, the sample can be considered negative for ringworm.

PRESERVING THE SAMPLES

If it is not possible to examine the sample immediately, they may be stored until required. It may also be necessary to send the sample to an external laboratory for analysis in which case appropriate storage will also be required. It is important that samples that are not going to be examined immediately are not allowed to dry out. Potassium hydroxide or liquid paraffin may be used as the lubricant. With the exception of smears, it is not advisable to send prepared microscope slides through the post as the sample is most likely to slip off the slide by the time it reaches its destination. Samples from skin scrapes can be placed into a 5 or 20 ml sterile universal sample pot along with the blade and sent to the laboratory. Always label the pot properly stating that a blade is in the pot to avoid any accidents. Samples of ear wax can be kept until ready or sent to the lab by cutting the cotton bud so that the piece with the sample on it, fits into a 5 or 20 ml universal sample pot. Special slide holders are available to send microscope slides in the post.

FURTHER READING

Bush, B.M (1975) *Veterinary Laboratory Manual*. Heineman, Oxford.

Bistner, S.I. & Ford, R.B. (1995) *Handbook of Veterinary Procedures and Emergency Treatment*, 6th edn. WB Saunders Company, London.

SECTION 7
EMERGENCY CARE AND FIRST AID

CHAPTER 39

INITIAL ASSESSMENT

Under the Veterinary Surgeons Act 1966 veterinary nurses may render first aid in an emergency for the purpose of saving a life or relieving pain or suffering in an animal. According to the guidelines from the Royal College of Veterinary Surgeons this is restricted to what is necessary to save an animal's life or stop pain or suffering until the veterinary surgeon can be contacted. It is therefore essential that qualified and listed nurses have the expertise and competence to carry out first aid procedures appropriate to the needs of the patients and that they are fully aware of all procedures that may be rendered in an emergency situation to fulfil the aims of first aid.

These notes list the action veterinary nurses should take in the event of being responsible for an emergency case arriving at the clinic.

AIMS OF FIRST AID

- Preservation of life
- Prevention of suffering
- Prevention of the deterioration of the patient's condition
- Relief of acute conditions

RULES

- Do not panic
- Maintain airway
- Control haemorrhage
- Contact the veterinary surgeon ASAP!

TELEPHONE CALLS – WHAT TO ASK

- Nature of injury and extent of injury
- Time of incident
- Breed, age, sex of animal
- Current veterinary treatment; diabetic? cardiac? epileptic?
- Caller's/owner's name, address and contact telephone number
- Their estimated time of arrival

Above all, calm and reassure the caller.

ADVICE TO CALLERS FOR HANDLING AND TRANSPORTATION OF THE INJURED ANIMAL

- Avoid further dangers to the animal or the caller (warn on-coming traffic, approach the animal carefully) – shocked and injured animals can become aggressive.
- Is the animal breathing? Clear airway, pulling tongue forward and removing debris from the mouth if possible without putting their hand in the animal's mouth, gently extend the neck unless there is obvious trauma.
- Control haemorrhage – apply constant pressure to affected area using material that is as clean as possible.
- Keep the animal warm using coats, blankets, etc.
- Advise caller about moving the animal – use a coat, blanket or board to make a stretcher following a road traffic accident (RTA) or multiple trauma.
- Use an aerated box or cat basket for cats and small dogs.
- Ensure the animal is secure and unable to escape.
- Keep the animal as immobile as possible ensuring the traumatised area is uppermost.
- Calm and reassure the animal.

PREPARATION AT THE VETERINARY CLINIC

- Inform all other veterinary staff of the nature of the accident
- Prepare kennelling – blankets and heat pads
- Prepare equipment for intravenous fluid therapy – warm fluids
- Prepare oxygen administration equipment
- Prepare emergency drugs

- Ensure X-ray developing machine is switched on

EXAMINATION OF THE PATIENT ON ARRIVAL AT THE CLINIC

A *Check and clear airway*: pull tongue forward, remove debris using swabs or suction, perform tracheotomy or intubate if necessary, perform Heimlich manoeuvre if necessary

B *Check breathing*: institute artificial respiration if necessary. If the animal is breathing, observe respiratory pattern – is inspiratory distress present? Evidence of obstruction; cover open wounds to throat or chest

C *Check circulation*: is there a heartbeat? If not start cardiopulmonary resuscitation (CPR)
- Is femoral or peripheral pulse palpable?
- Take core body temperature and take steps to maintain normothermia
- Control haemorrhage, cover open wounds using pressure with sterile dressing
- Administer intravenous fluids
- Relieve pain
- Temporarily immobilise fractures by keeping the animal in lateral recumbency, place animals with suspected spinal cord injuries on boards
- Perform an initial physical examination to assess the degree of injury using the mnemonic below

A CRASH PLAN to evaluate the patient

A   Airway – examine oral cavity, pharynx and neck
C   Cardiovascular system – monitor and record heart rate, pulse rate and quality
R   Respiratory system – observe respiratory movements, monitor and record respiratory rate and depth
A   Abdomen – examine and note any bruises, punctures and protrusions
S   Spine – neurological examination
H   Head – examine all parts, eyes, ears, nose, teeth and mouth
P   Pelvis
L   Limbs – examine for evidence of fractures, wounds
A   Arteries
N   Nerves – check reflexes to assess level of consciousness; pedal withdrawal reflex, pupillary and palpebral reflexes

MONITORING THE CRITICAL CARE PATIENT

Depending on the severity of the patients' condition, monitoring may be performed from anything from three times an hour to three times a day. The details should be recorded accurately so that trends may be noted.

DEMEANOUR

Whether the patient is bright and alert or lethargic, depressed and unresponsive. It is important to recognise whether a patient is normally quiet or whether it is a result of the condition.

TEMPERATURE

An increase in the animal's body temperature may indicate infection whilst a decrease may indicate shock. Check the extremities (paws and ears) to see if they feel cold. This may indicate poor peripheral perfusion often seen in cardiac disease.

PULSE

Measurement of the pulse gives an indication of the heart rate. Remember to check peripheral pulses as well as central pulse. This will give an idea of how good the circulation is.

RESPIRATION

Record the rate as well as the depth and rhythm. Does the animal require assisted ventilation or oxygen?

MUCOUS MEMBRANE COLOUR

The colour of the mucous membrane can give an indication of various conditions. Cyanotic colour and tachypnoea indicates hypoxia. A pale colour indicates shock, anaemia, or haemorrhage. Yellow mucous membranes indicate hepatic dysfunction.

CAPILLARY REFILL TIME

A prolonged capillary refill time indicates poor peripheral perfusion. Normal time should be less than 2 seconds.

URINE OUTPUT

In critical care patients, urine monitoring is important to assess kidney function. Closed urinary catheterisation ensures accurate recording. Assessment of urination without catheterisation or cystocentesis is less accurate but a record should be made of the number of times the animal has urinated, whether in its cage, litter tray or when taken outside.

APPETITE

Critical care patients are often inappetent and require assisted feeding techniques. Animals that are inappetent for long periods of time become cachexic, not only losing weight but also muscle mass as the body tries to assimilate energy from its own sources.

EMERGENCY CARE

CHAPTER 40

EMERGENCY PROCEDURES

It is important that the veterinary nurse is able to carry out various essential emergency procedures.

CARDIOPULMONARY RESUSCITATION (CPR)

Cardiopulmonary arrest is the cessation of ventilation and effective circulation. Irreversible brain damage starts to occur after 3 minutes without an oxygen supply and it is described as a 'three minute emergency'. The VN must be fully competent in the actions that must be taken in order for CPR to be effective. There is no time to consult manuals and it is obviously not a task that can be practised easily.

The main factors that control the degree of success include:

- Preventing the factors that predispose animals to cardiac arrest
- Recognising the signs of cardiac arrest
- Performing the appropriate CPR techniques in the correct sequence

FACTORS PREDISPOSING ANIMALS TO CARDIAC ARREST

If VNs are aware of the various causes of cardiac arrest they will not only be more likely to take care when nursing these high-risk patients but also more likely to take appropriate steps to prevent the situation developing into arrest.

- Drugs (e.g. anaesthetic drug overdose, digoxin, etc.)
- Toxins (e.g. endotoxin release during sepsis depresses cardiac function)
- Hypoxia
- Hypovolaemia/hypotension

- Acid–base imbalances (extremes in blood pH affect myocardial irritability and contractility)
- Electrolyte imbalances (abnormal potassium levels produce heart function changes)
- Extremes of temperature (changes seen with hypothermia dramatically increase risk of cardiac arrest)

SIGNS OF CARDIAC ARREST

- No pulse
- No heart beat
- Grey/cyanotic mucous membranes
- Dilated pupils, eye centrally fixed
- Increased CRT
- No respiratory movements or agonal gasps
- No bleeding at surgical site
- ECG – asystole, ventricular fibrillation or electromechanical dissociation.

Action

- The '3-minute emergency'. After 3 minutes irreversible brain damage may occur
- Carry out A B C procedure
- Inform VS: *note time*

It is necessary to clarify whether to commence CPR in the first place as it is a costly procedure and takes time and expertise. Several trained personnel are required throughout the resuscitation procedure to attend directly to the animal and also to fetch things and set up equipment. High-risk cases should therefore be discussed at the time of admission to the hospital or before surgery and those where CPR is not to be carried out should be identified. (NFR – *Not For Resuscitation* or DNR – *Do Not Resuscitate* signs can be placed on kennels of those cases when appropriate.) For those cases where CPR is indicated, it is essential that the arrest is identified as soon as it has happened and then appropriately acted upon straight away. Remember that this is a '3-minute emergency'.

EMERGENCY CARE

A – Airway

- Clear airway – remove mucous and debris, pull tongue forward
- Intubate

B – Breathing

- Intubate and ventilate with 100% oxygen
- One ventilation is given every 3–5 chest compressions (10–20 breaths per minute)

or

- Twice per 15 compressions if CPR is being performed by one person
- If intubation is not possible, then mouth to nose resuscitation is necessary (wear face mask or cover nose with swab)

C – Circulation – CHEST COMPRESSIONS

- 80–120 per minute
- Animal in right lateral recumbency, sandbag under thorax
- Compress over 6th intercostal space
- Use force appropriate to the size of the animal
- Ventilate every 3rd to 5th compression
- Hold compression for a brief time to maximise elimination of blood from the heart
- Feel for pulse

D – Drugs
Administer drugs under VS supervision. Possible drugs are:

- Adrenaline – stimulates sinus rhythm, increases contractility, and constricts peripheral vessels. Give intravenously or intracardiac.
- Lignocaine – if heart is fibrillating slows heart rate down.
- Sodium bicarbonate – to treat acidosis.

The use of each drug during CPR is dependent on the abnormality and ECG readings. The drugs can be administered by the following routes, in order of preference:

- Cranial vena cava (via a jugular catheter).

- Intratracheal (squirted into the trachea via a long catheter, through and beyond the endotracheal tube). It should be noted that higher doses than normal are required and the drugs should be added to 0.6 ml/kg of sterile saline.
- Intraosseous.
- Peripheral veins (slow reaction to drugs given by this route).
- Intracardiac (high potential hazards including intramyocardial injection, inducing fibrillation and pneumothorax).

Have a chart available with calculated drug doses for animals in increments of 2–5 kg

E – Electrocardiogram
Set up ECG

F – Fluids
Set up I/V line (crystalloid or colloid). The aim of fluid administration is to increase the circulating blood volume quickly. For this reason, colloids are the fluid of choice and should be injected as rapidly as possible by syringe at a volume of 25 ml/kg (cats) and 50 ml/kg (dogs). If colloids are not available, compound sodium lactate (Hartmann's) can be given at the same rate by squeezing the bag. After the initial infusion, fluids can be administered at a shock rate of 20 ml/kg/hour.

Signs of effective CPR

- Palpation of a femoral pulse during cardiac compression
- Constriction of the pupil
- Improvement in the colour of the mucous membranes
- Ventro-medial rotation of the eye
- ECG changes

Signs of continued improvement include

- Return of spontaneous respiration
- Return of palpebral eye reflex
- Vocalisation
- Lacrimation
- Return of movement, righting reflexes

INTRAVENOUS CATHETERISATION

Gaining venous access is one of the most important procedures in emergency care. Drugs and fluids can then be administered as necessary. Table 40.1 lists catheter sizes.

EQUIPMENT REQUIRED

- Clippers with number 40 or 50 blade
- Cleansing swabs (chlorhexidine scrub or other appropriate surgical soap)
- Swab soaked with isopropyl alcohol
- Cotton wool or gauze swabs
- 2.5 cm adhesive tape cut to lengths that will encircle catheterisation area
- Padding bandage material
- Conforming bandage
- Scissors
- Syringe containing 2 ml heparinised saline
- Appropriate size/type catheter (see Table 40.1)
- T-connector, 3-way tap or bung

CEPHALIC CATHETERISATION

Method:

(1) Collect the equipment and flush the T-connector, 3-way tap or bung with heparinised saline.
(2) Ensure the patient is adequately restrained.
(3) Clip a small square over the cephalic vein.
(4) Aseptically prepare the site with antiseptic solution and spirit.
(5) Ask the assistant to raise the vein.
(6) Identify the vein without touching the site. Stabilise the vein and insert the catheter with the bevel facing upwards.

Table 40.1 Catheter sizes.

Animal	Cephalic catheter	Jugular catheter
Cat or dog less than 10 kg	22–24 gauge	20–22 gauge
Medium-sized dog	20–22 gauge	18–20 gauge
Large dog	18–20 gauge	14–18 gauge

(7) As the catheter enters the vein, blood will appear in the hub of the catheter.

(8) Hold the stylet and advance the catheter into the vein up to the hub.

(9) Ask the assistant to place their thumb 2–3 cm above the catheter entry site to prevent blood flow.

(10) Remove the stylet and attach the connector (T-connector or 3-way tap).

(11) Secure the catheter by placing a strip of tape under the hub of the catheter then around the leg and back over the top of the hub. Further strips of tape may be placed around the connector.

(12) A dressing (Opsite™) may be placed over the catheter site to prevent infection.

(13) The catheter should then be covered with a padding layer and outer cohesive bandage.

JUGULAR CATHETERISATION TECHNIQUE (USING A 'THROUGH-THE-NEEDLE' JUGULAR CATHETER)

Method:

(1) Collect all necessary equipment and flush the T-connector with heparinised saline.

(2) Assistant restrains the animal in lateral recumbency, extending head to enable access to the jugular.

(3) A small sandbag placed under the neck will enhance visualisation and catheterisation of the jugular.

(4) Clip hair over the jugular area approximately 10 × 10 cm.

(5) Wash hands.

(6) Aseptically prepare the site using surgical soap.

(7) Rinse soap suds off with swab soaked in isopropyl alcohol.

(8) Raise the vein by applying pressure with the thumb to the jugular groove.

(9) Hold the needle firmly in one hand, and insert through the skin in a caudal direction toward the thoracic inlet.

(10) Insert the needle through the skin before attempting to enter into the vein.

(11) Stabilise the jugular vein with the free hand and with one sharp movement, pass the catheter into the vein.

(12) When blood appears in the hub and lumen of the catheter advance the catheter 1 cm further.

EMERGENCY CARE

(13) Still holding the catheter in the right hand, thread the catheter into the vein by pushing it through the metal needle within the plastic sleeve.
(14) Disconnect the plastic sleeve from the needle.
(15) Take the metal needle out of the skin and place the protective plastic needle guard over the needle and snap closed.
(16) Place injection cap on to catheter.
(17) Flush catheter with heparinised saline.

Useful tips

In thick-skinned animals, animals in shock or dehydration, it may be advantageous to make a nick through the skin just above the vein to help visualise and catheterise the vein more easily. The skin is pulled away from the vein and a small cut is made in the skin using a 20 gauge needle or number 11 surgical blade. The catheter can then be inserted through the skin at this point.

Effective restraint of the patient is essential for successful catheter placement – take time to make the animal more at ease and provide lots of vocal reassurance.

If possible, try to place catheters before administration of sedatives such as acepromazine or medetomidine, which dramatically drop blood pressure thus making catheterisation more difficult.

Appropriate dilution of heparinised saline may be made by adding 0.1 ml of heparin (1:1000) to 100 ml of sterile saline.

THE HEIMLICH MANOEUVRE

For removal of an obstructive foreign body in the larynx.

(1) Suspend patient upside down by the hind legs
(2) Large dogs may be hung over a table or fence
(3) Administer sharp punch to abdominal wall just above the xiphisternum and towards the diaphragm
(4) The patient should cough and expel the foreign body

If the obstruction is not dislodged – an emergency tracheotomy may be required.

TRACHEOTOMY

To relieve upper respiratory obstructions in order to alleviate asphyxiation.

In an emergency situation any sharp instrument can be used to make the tracheotomy hole. A large bore needle (14–16 gauge) can be inserted between two cartilage rings to provide ventilatory access.

Method:

(1) Damp the hair over the trachea with surgical spirit
(2) Make an incision caudal to the larynx (between 3rd and 4th tracheal ring)
(3) Insert a small endotracheal tube (5 mm noncuffed) directing downwards towards the lungs
(4) Oxygen may then be administered

Usually this is a temporary measure until the obstruction is removed.

STOMACH TUBING FOR GASTRIC DILATION

It is important to try to relieve the excess gas that builds up as quickly as possible.

(1) Measure the tube from the caudal end of the ribs to the nose.
(2) Place a mouth gag or a role of bandage in the animal's mouth so that the tube can be fed through the middle.
(3) Lubricate the end of the tube and gently insert into the oesophagus allowing the animal to swallow.
(4) As soon as the tube enters the stomach air and stomach contents will come back up the tube.
(5) If the stomach is twisted it may not be possible to pass the tube in which case surgery is necessary.
(6) After the stomach is decompressed it may be lavaged several times with water or a water and charcoal solution.
(7) Observe the animal closely for further signs of gastric distension.
(8) A measuring tape or piece of nonconforming bandage may be used to measure the abdominal circumference at frequent intervals to check for enlargement.

EMERGENCY CARE

MANUAL POSITIVE PRESSURE VENTILATION

INDICATIONS

- Resuscitation in the event of respiratory/cardiac arrest
- During intrathoracic surgery
- Following administration of neuromuscular blocking agents
- Respiratory inadequacy

EQUIPMENT

- Intubated animal
- 'Ambu' Resuscitator self-inflating bag (see Fig. 40.1)

or

- Suitable anaesthetic breathing system, e.g. Ayres T-piece with Jackson-Rees modification (open-ended bag) or Bains
- Oxygen supply – room air (approximately 20% oxygen) or preferably oxygen supply (anaesthetic machine)

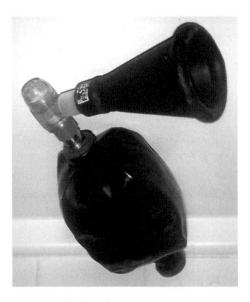

Fig. 40.1   Resuscitator self-inflating bag.

Rate
Should mimic the animal's normal respiration rate:

- Dogs: 10–20 breaths per minute
- Cats: 20–30 breaths per minute

Tidal volume

- 10–20 ml/kg
- Should be sufficient to produce good chest movements (excessive pressure must be avoided to prevent lung damage)

Pattern
The inspiratory phase should last only about one-third of the time of the total ventilatory cycle; a short inflation followed by a longer expiratory pause. This facilitates venous return. A time ratio of 1:2 is recommended. For example, for an animal receiving a rate of 20 breaths per minute, a 1 second inflation is followed by 2 seconds rest.

TECHNIQUE

(1) Allow the bag on the circuit to inflate by partially blocking the open end of the bag or temporarily closing the over-expiratory valve
(2) Inflate the lungs by squeezing the bag – chest wall movement should be more obvious than in normal breathing
(3) Release the open end of bag or open valve to allow expiration

In cats it is advisable to keep the endotracheal tube uncuffed to avoid over-inflating the lungs.

OXYGEN THERAPY

Oxygen therapy is required when there is inadequate tissue oxygenation (hypoxia). This can occur due to dyspnoea or circulatory failure (shock). It is important to remember that hypoxic animals do not necessarily show clinical signs until things are extremely severe and for this reason, oxygen therapy should be considered for any patient with reduced lung volume or poor peripheral perfusion. Do not wait until an animal exhibits signs associated with hypoxia (e.g. dyspnoea, cyanosis, cold extremities, cardiac rate changes, etc.) before starting therapy.

The aim of oxygen therapy is to increase the amount of oxygen in the blood by increasing the arterial oxygen tension and this can be achieved using the following methods at the stated flow rates and administration techniques. The condition and demeanour of the patient need to be considered and the method of administering oxygen should take into account the most appropriate method for the patient.

OXYGEN MASK

Oxygen masks are good for emergency and short-term use. However, conscious patients are often distressed by the mask, which in turn causes further respiratory distress.

- A face mask is attached to a nonrebreathing anaesthetic system (e.g. Bain system) and connected to an oxygen source such as an anaesthetic machine
- A high flow rate of 10 l/min or more is required to prevent carbon dioxide build up inside the mask
- The mask is fitted over mouth and nose of the patient but not so that it is airtight (exhaled carbon dioxide must escape into room air)

OXYGEN CAGE

Oxygen cages are useful for smaller animals and many cages or incubators have the advantage of being heated and humidified. However, it can be difficult to observe and manage the patient effectively and each time the door is opened, the oxygen concentration will drop significantly.

- A high flow rate of 10 l/min of oxygen is required initially to flush out residual nitrogen in the cage
- This can then be reduced to about 5 l/min for maintenance
- The cage should be warmed to 18–21°C (65–70°F) in most situations

HIGH FLOW-BY

High flow-by oxygen delivery is useful in emergencies and when the animal is open-mouth breathing.

- An anaesthetic system tubing (e.g. Magill Circuit) is placed by patient's face
- High flow rates of 10 l/min or more are required

INTRATRACHEAL CATHETER

This method is particularly useful in animals too large to fit into an oxygen cage, but it is sometimes difficult to restrain the animal for placement of the catheter without causing further stress. It is particularly useful when there is laryngeal/pharyngeal obstruction.

- A 14 gauge through-the-needle intravenous catheter is placed aseptically into the trachea between the tracheal rings
- The catheter is attached to the oxygen supply via a large, male urinary catheter
- Oxygen may be administered at a rate of 100 ml/kg/min
- Oxygen must be humidified

NASAL CATHETER

Nasal catheters are usually well tolerated by the patient and it suitable for long-term use. However, they take time to set up and so are no good for emergency use.

- Apply topical local anaesthetic drops into the nose of the patient
- Insert a soft 5 FG or 8 FG feeding tube in as far as the midnasal region via one nostril
- Extend the tube up the face between the eyes and attach to the skin on the top of the head (shave a small area) using either sutures or glue
- It is advisable to fit an Elizabethan collar to prevent patient interference
- The oxygen must be humidified
- Flow rates of 50–100 ml/kg/min should be used depending on the size of the tube

PLASTIC HOOD

A large clear plastic bag placed over the patient's head is an efficient and well-tolerated method of administering oxygen in an emergency.

- One corner of the bag must be cut to allow the oxygen tubing to pass through
- Tape is used to seal the bag around the tube
- The bottom of the bag should be left open to allow exhaled carbon dioxide to escape
- Flow rates of 200 ml/kg/min can be used

ELIZABETHAN COLLAR

An inexpensive and easily set up system, which is well tolerated, especially by cats.

- 'Cling film' is placed over the front of an Elizabethan collar
- A small gap must be left at the bottom to allow removal of exhaled carbon dioxide
- A small tube is taped to the inside of the collar and connects with the oxygen supply unit
- Flow rates of 2–4 l/min can be used

NOTES ON HUMIDIFICATION OF OXYGEN

In the normal patient, air passing through the airways is warmed, moistened and filtered by the epithelial cells of the nasopharynx. Humidification is essential when oxygen therapy is being delivered using a system which bypasses the patient's own humidification system. Administer the oxygen by passing the flow through a bottle of warmed saline.

CHAPTER 41

FLUID THERAPY

FLUID THERAPY SOLUTIONS

WHICH SOLUTION?

There is a tendency to use the same solution for fluid therapy no matter what the cause. Generally this is not a problem in the short term as the main goal is to correct the fluid deficit. Hartmann's is a good choice for most conditions as it contains electrolytes in very similar concentrations to those in ECF. For each case, consider which electrolytes are being lost and replace like with like. In conditions where urinary output has failed (e.g. urethral obstruction, acute renal failure, bladder rupture), metabolites and electrolytes which are normally excreted in the urine accumulate in the body. This will also lead to an imbalance.

CLASSIFICATION OF SOLUTIONS

- Crystalloids
- Colloids
- Whole blood

CRYSTALLOID SOLUTIONS

A group of sodium-based electrolyte fluids. Crystalloids enter the extracellular fluid and equilibrate with other fluid compartments to restore fluid balance.

Most commonly used crystalloids are similar to plasma in composition.

Normal saline 0.9% – isotonic

- Contains sodium and chloride

- Useful for replacing/maintaining blood volume during anaesthesia and surgery
- The high level of sodium makes this fluid unsuitable for long-term maintenance
- Useful for gastric vomiting

Compound sodium lactate (Hartmann's) – isotonic

- Contains sodium, chloride, potassium, bicarbonate and calcium
- Useful in a wide range of diseases; pyometra, diarrhoea, metabolic acidosis, peri-operative fluid support
- The electrolyte concentration is similar to plasma

Dextrose 4% and saline 0.18%

- This solution is mainly water with a small amount of sodium and chloride
- Useful for maintenance and primary water loss
- For long-term maintenance, potassium should be added

5% Glucose

- Essentially water with approximately 50 mg/ml glucose added to make it isotonic
- Used for primary water loss and to help correct hypoglycaemia

Ringers solution

- Contains sodium, chloride, potassium and calcium
- Used for mainly water and electrolyte losses; e.g. pyometra with vomiting

COLLOID SOLUTIONS

Colloids are a group of fluids containing large molecules that will remain in the intravascular space. They help to expand the circulating volume of the blood – 'plasma expanders'. They also help to increase the osmotic pressure preventing further plasma loss into cells and interstitial spaces.

Dextrans (70 or 40 – indicates molecular weight)

- Artificial colloid solutions with a high molecular weight. Not used routinely in UK
- Crystalloids should be administered at same time to prevent cellular dehydration

Gelatins

- Straw-coloured isotonic solutions derived from gelatin
  - e.g. Gelofusin and Haemaccel
- These products should be stored at room temperature
- If they are to be warmed they must be heated in a water bath (*do not* microwave – this will destroy the protein constituents)
- Remain in the circulation for approximately 5 hours

WHOLE BLOOD

Should be used in cases of:

- Severe haemorrhage
- Severe anaemia
- Blood clotting disorders

BLOOD PRODUCTS

Plasma
Plasma may be separated from the cellular part of blood and administered to replace plasma proteins. It also minimises the risk of transfusion reactions.

Red cells
Packed red cells may also be given to replace cell loss. Administered simultaneously with saline solution.

Table 41.1 summarises fluid therapy solutions.

CALCULATING RATES OF ADMINISTRATION

A fluid plan needs to be worked out in order to calculate total fluid requirements. Existing deficits, maintenance and continuing losses all need to be taken into account.

Table 41.1 Summary of fluid therapy solutions.

Solution	Crystalloid/colloid	Osmolarity	Composition	Indications
0.9% Normal saline	Crystalloid	Isotonic	Na, Cl	Loss of chloride: e.g. vomiting and general ECF replacement
Compound sodium lactate (Hartmann's)	Crystalloid	Isotonic	Na, Cl, K, HCO_3, Ca	Use in cases of acidosis: e.g. diarrhoea and general ECF replacement
0.18% NaCl and 4% dextrose	Crystalloid	Isotonic	Na, Cl, dextrose	Good maintenance fluid
Ringer's solution	Crystalloid	Isotonic	Na, Cl, K, Ca	Use in alkalosis: e.g. persistent vomiting
5% Dextrose	Crystalloid	Isotonic	Dextrose	Water losses
Haemaccel/gelofusin	Colloid	Isotonic	Na, Cl and gelatins	Restoration of circulating volume
Plasma	Colloid	Isotonic	Plasma	Restoration of circulating volume
Whole blood	Colloid	Isotonic	Whole blood	Replacement of blood, plasma, platelets and colloids
Dextrans	Colloid	Hypertonic	Na, Cl, dextrose	Restore circulating volume

1. REHYDRATION

The amount of fluid required to correct the existing deficit. This may be estimated in the following ways:

(1) Assessing from clinical signs how dehydrated the animal is (5%, 10%, etc.).

Multiply the percentage dehydration by the bodyweight and then by a factor of 10 to estimate the volume of fluid in mls required.

Example
A 20 kg dog is 5% dehydrated.

$20 \times 5 \times 10 = 1000\,ml$

Therefore approximately *1 litre* is required to replace the existing deficit.

(2) Assessing fluid loss from an increase in PCV.

Example
A 20 kg animal has a PCV of 55%.

$(55\% - 45\%) \times 20 \times 10 = 2000\,\text{ml}$

(3)   Assessing loss from history from owner.

Losses from vomiting and diarrhoea, etc., multiplied by the number of days.

Example
    A 20 kg dog has had no food or water for 3 days and has been vomiting three times daily for 3 days.

3 days vomiting at 4 ml/kg/vomit = 720 ml

2. MAINTENANCE

Maintenance equals 50 ml/kg bodyweight/24 hours.
    For example, maintenance for a 20 kg dog:

$50 \times 20 = 1000\,\text{ml}/24\,\text{hours}$

3. CONTINUING LOSSES

As well as rehydration and maintenance fluids, compensation must also be made for continuing losses through vomiting and diarrhoea.
    Estimated losses (in ml) are added to the fluid plan.

Example
    A cat vomits approximately 20 ml of fluid and excretes approximately 40 ml of watery diarrhoea daily.
    Therefore 60 ml of fluid must be added to the 24 hour fluid plan.

THE WHOLE FLUID PLAN

A 40 kg dog is estimated to be 8% dehydrated. The dog is vomiting approximately 400 ml each day. What will the fluid requirements be for the first 24 hours?

(1) Rehydration	3200 ml
(2) Maintenance	2000 ml
(3) Continuing loss	400 ml
Total	5600 ml/24 hours

RATE OF FLUID REPLACEMENT

Factors that affect the rate of infusion.

- Rate of loss
- Health of patient
- Type of fluid
- Ongoing losses

Blood volume in adult animal = 90 ml/kg
Therefore:
The *maximum rate* of infusion of crystalloids should not exceed 90 ml/kg/hour for 1 hour only.
It is possible to administer 20–30 ml/kg/hour for less severe dehydration or administration of colloids.

HOW FAST? WORKING OUT THE DRIP RATE

If the maintenance rate is known – the VN needs to know what the drip rate is going to be.
Different giving sets administer different amounts of drops per ml. For example, paediatric sets (burette) deliver 60 drops/ml, whereas most other sets deliver 20 drops/ml.
Paediatric or burette sets are more accurate and should be used on cats and small dogs to prevent over-infusion.
Method:

(1) Calculate maintenance requirements
(2) Divide the total by 24 to obtain amount in hours
(3) Then divide by 60 to obtain ml per minute
(4) Multiply this figure by the drip factor (either 20 drops per ml or 60 drops per ml)
(5) This will give the number of drops per minute

In summary:

total amount required in 24 hours divided by 24 = hourly rate

hourly rate/60 = minute rate

minute rate × administration drip factor (e.g. 20) = drops per minute

Calculations

A 15 kg dog requires 1500 ml over 24 hours. What rate should the fluids be set at using an administration set that delivers 20 drops/ml?

Answer:

$$1500/24 = 62.5 \, ml/hour$$

$$62.5/60 = 1.04 \, ml/minute$$

$$1.04 \times 20 = 20.8 \, drops/minute$$

which is the equivalent of 1 drop every 3 seconds.

EQUIPMENT AND TECHNIQUE

Ensure all equipment is prepared before placing the intravenous catheter. Prefill the T-connector with heparinised saline (one unit heparin per ml of 0.9% saline), cut lengths of securing tape and warm the fluids to body temperature. Fluid pumps are becoming more popular, and these provide accurate dosing of fluid. Syringe pumps are useful in small pets to deliver lower volumes.

Method:

(1) Set up fluid bag and giving set
   - Check expiry date.
   - Warm the fluids to body heat.
   - Remove outer package.
   - Break seal to giving port and open giving set bag and close off the giving set regulator.
   - Insert giving set into bag (do not contaminate the set).
   - Squeeze the drip chamber to fill half full.
   - Open the regulator and allow fluids to fill up giving set tubing. There should be *no* bubbles in the tubing.
(2) Select suitable gauge catheter for one of the following veins
   - Cephalic
   - Saphenous
   - Jugular
   - Medial femoral
(3) Clip site and aseptically prepare it
   - Take care not to cause clipper rash

- Use skin preparation solutions to thoroughly cleanse skin

(4) Introduce catheter into the vein
  - Assistant to raise appropriate vein
  - Stabilise vein with thumb or tense skin
  - Do not touch catheter barrel
  - Use new catheter if kinking or contamination occurs
  - Insert with bevel facing upwards
  - Advance catheter half way into vein (should feel a 'pop' and venous blood should appear in the hub)
  - Stabilise the stylet
  - With other hand – gently advance the catheter into the vein

(5) Attach T-connector or 3-way tap
  - Already filled with heparinised saline

(6) Flush catheter with heparinised saline
  - To keep catheter patent, flush every 6 hours with heparinised saline

(7) Secure catheter with tape
  - Place first piece of tape beneath catheter and around the limb, ensure the catheter is secure

(8) Connect fluid supply
  - Ensure distal end of giving set remains sterile

(9) Apply bandage over the site to cover the catheter and giving set
  - Examine the site daily for evidence of infection or swelling

MONITORING THE PATIENT

- Check fluid is flowing at the correct rate
- Flush line with heparinised saline if blocked
- Do not flush with force – may need to change catheter
- Extend animals leg – may be a positional blockage
- Prevent patient interference

CENTRAL VENOUS PRESSURE

Central venous pressure (CVP) is a method of measuring venous blood pressure in the anterior vena cava. The measurement indicates the heart's ability to pump venous return and the adequacy of the circulating blood volume. It aids clinical evaluation of patients with reduced blood volume and impaired cardiac function and is of particular benefit in hypovolaemic, geriatric and surgical cases.

The CVP measurement is the first parameter to change when the circulation is compromised and the last parameter to return to normal during recovery and it is for this reason that it makes it a valuable guide to the animal's response to treatment. Much more so than other physical signs such as temperature, pulse quality and mucous membrane colour.

Normal values

There is no absolute normal value for CVP, and as seen from the normal values shown below, there is a wide range in the cat and dog. What is more important and of greater value, is to obtain frequent readings and thus establish a trend. The findings can be recorded and an appropriate response to increases or decreases implemented as necessary.

Normal CVP range $= 0$–5 cm of H_2O

Increases above the normal range indicate expanded blood volume, either due to fluid replacement being administered too quickly or the heart/kidney's inability to cope with the infusion. Increases above 15 cm of H_2O indicate circulatory overload and all fluid administration should be stopped.

Decreases in CVP indicate that blood volume replacement is indicated or that the current fluid administration rate is inadequate.

MEASUREMENT OF CENTRAL VENOUS PRESSURE

Equipment:

- Jugular catheter of appropriate size for the animal
- Metric ruler
- 3-way taps
- 500 ml sodium chloride 0.9%
- Administration set
- Extension sets
- Tape

Method:

(1) Clip and aseptically prepare jugular site.
(2) Place jugular catheter and secure in place.

(3) Connect 3-way tap to the catheter.

(4) Connect an I/V set-up of the normal saline to one port of the 3-way tap.

(5) To the other port of the 3-way tap, connect an extension set, which is taped to the metric ruler.

(6) The '0' on the metric rule should be taped to the table so that it lies in line with right atrium in the animal (roughly level with the manubrium when the animal is in lateral recumbency).

(7) Fill the CVP manometer line (extension set) until it exceeds the 15 cm mark.

(8) Switch the 3-way tap so that the jugular is now open to the manometer tube.

(9) The level will fall and stabilise at the CVP.

(10) Read this measurement against the ruler and record.

Commercial manometers are available and can be used in place of the improvised technique identified above. However, these are relatively expensive and are not widely used in practice. The method shown above is an inexpensive and extremely effective way of obtaining a CVP measurement.

BLOOD TRANSFUSIONS

Due to the increasing specialisation of small animal veterinary practice, the need and frequency for administration of whole blood has risen dramatically. Blood transfusions are integral to the support care of critically ill and anaemic patients and can save the lives of many patients. It is relatively easy to find suitable blood donors, and many practices have a donor list of clients who are happy to lend their dog or cat when required. The collection, cross-matching and administration of blood is, however, a time consuming and labour-intensive process and requires a certain amount of expertise and specialised equipment. The VN must be competent in all aspects of practical administration and confident at monitoring the patient receiving the blood.

AIMS OF BLOOD TRANSFUSION

- To restore oxygen-carrying capacity of blood
- Replace various blood components (plasma proteins, platelets, clotting factors)

Main indications
- Haemorrhage: acute, chronic and immune based
- Haemolysis: e.g. blood parasites
- Reduced RBC production: e.g. bone marrow disease
- Thrombocytopaenia: destruction of own platelets
- Coagulopathies: e.g. Von Willebrand's disease
- Hypoproteinaemia: loss of protein – gastrointestinal disorders, burns, etc.

Anaemia is the main indication for a blood transfusion in veterinary practice. Patients with nonregenerative anaemia will benefit from a transfusion because the transfused RBCs last for approximately 30–60 days, providing life-saving time for diagnostic work-ups and initiation of appropriate treatments. Clinical evaluation of the patient is the determining factor in deciding whether a blood transfusion is to be performed. Any anaemic animal exhibiting signs of weakness, dyspnoea or a worsening of their condition in response to stress should be considered a candidate for transfusion.

Bear in mind that many patients do not exhibit marked clinical signs of anaemia until the latter stages of the disease and so it is essential that a PCV measurement is obtained in suspected cases.

It has been recommended that a transfusion should be administered if the patient shows clinical signs of anaemia and the PCV is less than 10%, or if there has been a rapid decrease in the PCV to less than 15–20%).

BLOOD COLLECTION – CHOOSING A DONOR

Table 41.2 shows which dogs and cats make suitable donors. *Note*:

- Greyhounds have a higher PCV (48–66%) therefore are very useful as donors
- Giant breeds may be able to give more than 1 unit

Table 41.2 Suitable dogs and cats for blood donation.

Dogs	Cats
> 25 kg	> 5kg
Healthy, wormed, vaccinated	Healthy, wormed, vaccinated
PCV > 40%	PCV > 35%
Calm temperament	Calm temperament

- A minimum of 4–6 weeks should be left in between each donation

BLOOD COLLECTION CONTAINERS

Dogs

Human collection bags provide 1 unit (450 ml blood + 50 ml anticoagulant) and contain anticoagulants to prevent clotting and to preserve the blood. They may be used for dogs over 25 kg. (If less than 450 ml is to be collected, a proportionate amount of anticoagulant should be removed from the bag.)

Anticoagulants used in human blood bags:

- CPDA (citrate-phosphate-dextrose-adenine) or
- ACD (acid-citrate-dextrose)

Cats

Blood for feline transfusion can be collected into a 50 ml syringe containing 7 ml of ACD or CPDA (withdrawn from a human blood collection bag). There should be 1.4 ml of anticoagulant to every 10 ml of blood.

AMOUNT TO TAKE

No more than 20% of blood volume should be obtained. As a general rule, up to 10% of a donor's blood can be taken without adverse effects on the donor. Up to 20% of blood volume can be obtained but intravenous fluids should be administered during and after collection. (Crystalloids given 2 × the amount of blood taken.)

Total blood volume = 90 ml/kg for dogs and 60 ml/kg for cats.

- Dogs = 22 ml/kg
- Cats = 15 ml/kg

METHOD OF COLLECTION

Find a quiet room and at least three people:

- Assistant to restrain animal
- Assistant to hold blood bag and mix the collected blood

- Person to carry out venipuncture

The owners may wish to stay with their animal and they may be useful to help restrain and calm the pet during the procedure.

(1) Sedate donor animal if necessary (avoid circulatory depressants such as medetomidine).

(2) Collect all necessary equipment; clippers, collection bag, alcohol swabs and surgical scrub, etc.

(3) Assistant to restrain donor for jugular venipuncture. (Giant breeds sitting on floor, smaller dogs sitting or in lateral recumbency on a table. Cats in lateral recumbency on table.)

(4) Clip and aseptically prepare site over jugular.

(5) Raise the jugular vein and aseptically place the blood bag needle into the jugular vein (or 21G butterfly catheter pre-filled with anticoagulant and attached to 50 ml syringe in cats).

(6) Hold the collection bag lower than animal (gravity enhances flow rates) or apply very gentle suction to the syringe (excess suction will collapse the vein).

(7) Second assistant gently agitates the bag or the operator inverts the syringe regularly throughout collection to thoroughly mix the blood with the anticoagulant.

(8) Check the bag periodically to ensure that the blood is still flowing.

(9) Continue until the desired quantity of blood is obtained. The bag can be weighed to find out approximate measurement because 1 ml of blood weighs roughly 1 g. (A full bag should weigh approximately 500 g.)

(10) Remove the jugular needle and the assistant should apply pressure for at least 5 minutes, over the venipuncture site to prevent a haematoma forming.

(11) Tie the collection bag tubing in several places along its length and label bag with the donor's name, date of collection, and date of expiry.

(12) Advise the owners to keep the donor animal calm for at least 30 minutes and rested for the remainder of the day. They should avoid putting a lead and collar on for as long as possible and can feed the animal after the procedure.

DONOR/RECIPIENT BLOOD MATCHING

Before transfusion is carried out, a cross-matching test or blood typing analysis should be carried out to ensure that the donor blood is compatible with the recipient's blood thereby reducing the likelihood of a transfusion reaction. Blood matching is especially vital in feline transfusion or second transfusions in dogs, because fatal reactions can occur if incompatible blood groups are mixed. Transfusion reactions due to blood mismatches are rare in most first-time blood transfusions in dogs, but the risk of a transfusion reactions are much higher for subsequent transfusions and so blood matching is again strongly recommended.

There are two methods of ensuring that donor and recipient blood is compatible:

- Blood typing
- Cross-matching

BLOOD TYPING

Dogs
There are eight different blood groups that have been identified in dogs: dog erythrocyte antigen (DEA). Ideal blood groups are DEA 1.1 (negative) and DEA 1.2 (negative), which account for approximately 40% of the dog population. These blood groups should ideally be used whenever possible in transfusions, because they do not produce antibodies against blood and can be used safely in dogs that have previously received blood transfusions.

Kits are available to detect DEA 1.1 blood type in dogs (*Rapid Vet H™ – Canine 1.1 DMS™*).

Cats
There are three blood groups in cats – A, B and AB.

- A group – most common, generally domestic short-hair and Siamese types
- B group – mainly domestic long-hair and exotics
- AB group – rare

Although blood type A is the most common, the frequency of types A and B varies geographically and among breeds. Like humans, cats have significant naturally occurring antibodies against the blood type antigen that they lack. It is essential that blood-typing or cross-matching be carried out first to prevent potential fatal reactions.

Kits are available to blood-type cats (*Rapid Vet H*™ – *Feline H, DMS*™)

CROSS-MATCHING

Cross-matching is a test that is performed to assess whether the donor and recipient serum antibodies will mix and not destroy each other. Blood samples must be obtained from both the donor and the recipient and collected into heparin and EDTA sample tubes. Samples of plasma and washed blood cells are mixed on slides and the samples examined for evidence of agglutination and possible haemolysis of the blood cells.

TRANSFUSION QUANTITIES

The aim of transfusion is to increase the recipient's PCV to above 20–30%. This should reverse the signs of anaemia and alleviate the life-threatening condition of the patient.

The following formula can be used to estimate the volume of blood needed for transfusion:

body weight (kg) × 90 × PCV desired-PCV of recipient/PCV of donor

Example
A 15 kg dog, has a PCV of 10% and the aim of transfusion is to get up to a PCV of 25%. The PCV of the donor dog is 40%

$$15 \times 90 \times (25-10)/40 = 506.25$$

Therefore, 500 ml of whole blood should be given to this patient to achieve the desired PCV.

METHOD OF ADMINISTRATION

Route
Cephalic or jugular vein via an intravenous or jugular catheter.

Temperature

Freshly collected blood will be at the correct temperature for immediate administration. Refrigerated blood will need to be warmed to body temperature (38°C) before administration. This should be achieved slowly to avoid clotting and red cell lysis. Blood warmers (waterbaths and dry heat blood warmers are available) or the administration set tubing can be placed in warm water to achieve this.

Administration sets

Normal fluid administration sets are not suitable. Many of them do not contain any filtering system so run the risk of allowing small clots to enter the circulation and sets that do contain filters tend to clog because the filters are too small for blood. Special blood administration sets are available for attachment to the blood bag and connection to the catheter, and these should be used in all cases.

Blood collected into syringes from cats should be transferred into a blood bag that has had the anticoagulant removed. This then enables a blood administration set to be attached in the normal way.

Speed of administration

- 2 ml/kg/hour for patients with heart disease or renal disease
- 5–10 ml/kg/hour for normovolaemic patients
- Up to 20 ml/kg/hour for hypovolaemic patients

MONITORING THE RECIPIENT

Before transfusion obtain and record:

- PCV
- Temperature, pulse and respiration rates. CRT and colour of mucous membranes

During transfusion the patient should be monitored constantly and vigilantly. In addition, you should:

- Monitor vital signs every 30 minutes
- Measure PCV half way through transfusion to check for haemolysis
- Observe for any evidence of a transfusion reaction

CLINICAL SIGNS OF TRANSFUSION REACTION

Transfusion reactions should be rare in cases where correctly matched blood has been administered. However, it is essential to be aware of the potential risk of any transfusion, be able to recognise the signs and act appropriately.

- Discomfort, crying
- Circling, tremors
- Facial oedema
- Urticaria
- Tachypnoea or dyspnoea
- Tachycardia or bradycardia
- Vomiting
- Increased temperature
- Collapse
- Haematuria

In the case of a transfusion reaction, stop the blood administration and contact the attending veterinary surgeon immediately. Set up and administer intravenous crystalloid therapy and administer supportive therapy as directed by the veterinary surgeon (e.g. corticosteroids, oxygen, antihistamines and adrenaline). Antihistamines and steroids are sometimes given prior to transfusion to help reduce minor reactions occurring.

Apart from mismatching of blood, other causes of transfusion reaction include:

- Bacterial contamination of donor blood
- Inappropriate rate of infusion (too fast)
- Inappropriate quantities of anticoagulant used
- Use of an administration set without a filter
- Old blood, or blood that has been incorrectly stored

STORAGE OF WHOLE BLOOD

All blood taken from a donor and not used immediately needs to be stored in a refrigerator at 4°C. The blood bags should be placed inside another plastic bag to avoid contamination of the fridge should spillage occur. Ensure all blood collected is labelled with the donor's details, date of collection and date of expiry. If the blood transfusion to the recipient is required for platelet replacement it should be used within 6 hours. For RBC replacement it should used within 4 weeks.

EMERGENCY CARE

CHAPTER 42

FIRST AID – THE A–Z OF SPECIFIC CONDITIONS

You may only render first aid in an emergency for the purpose of saving a life or relieving pain or suffering until the veterinary surgeon can be obtained. When questioned in an exam about what you should do in the event of a '... ...', the first thing you should say is *"Contact the veterinary surgeon."*

ABDOMINAL RUPTURE

Abdominal ruptures may be caused by road traffic accidents (RTAs), bites, gunshot wounds and following abdominal surgery. The abdominal viscera escape through a tear in the abdominal muscle wall and may become strangulated (blood supply to escaped viscera becomes compromised or totally cut off). The abdominal viscera may or may not be protruding through the skin. Occasionally, no external wound is seen, but the escaped viscera lies under the skin surface. In open wounds the abdominal viscera can be seen on the surface of the wound.

- **Clean the open wound and viscera** – use warmed sterile saline to remove gross dirt
- **Prevent damage and further contamination** of the exposed viscera
  - **Cover viscera** with a swab soaked in warm, sterile saline
  - Cover sterile swab with **cling film** or clean **plastic bag** to help prevent swab drying out
  - Apply **abdominal bandage**
- **Treat shock** and **constantly monitor** patient
- **Prevent self-trauma** – Elizabethan collar
- Check under bandage every 15 minutes to ensure that viscera are not being damaged by the abdominal bandage
- Prepare for surgery

ASPHYXIA (SUFFOCATION)

This can occur as a result of many conditions such as, airway foreign body, collapsed trachea, swelling of pharynx, poisoning, thoracic crushing injuries, inhalation of noxious fumes and gases, and pneumothorax. The first aid treatment of these specific conditions are covered, however, it is essential that you know the clinical signs of asphyxia and general first aid treatment.

Clinical signs include:

- **Air hunger** – gasping for air, open mouth breathing, exaggerated respiratory movements
- **Orthopnoea**
- **Tachypnoea**
- **Hyperaesthesia** – these patients are excitable, stressed and react dramatically to any stimulus
- **Cyanosis** – often not seen until situation is extremely severe and death occurs soon unless therapeutic action is taken immediately (carbon monoxide poisoning is an exception – mucous membranes become cherry red)
- **Tachycardia**

General treatment includes:

- Do not stress
- Handle as little as possible
- Place in quiet, dark room
- Reassure – being unable to breathe is a terrifying experience – calm and gently reassure the animal
- Remove cause of asphyxia
- Provide oxygen
- Treat shock
- Observe constantly (but this is probably one of the few occasions when you should not obtain frequent temperature and respiration rates – this just stresses the animal further)

BURNS

Common causes of burns include heat pads, electrical cords, house fires, ceramic hobs, chemicals and hair dryers. The full extent of the injury may not be evident for 2–3 weeks after the initial burn has occurred; however, if the burn area is evident or known, immediate first aid treatment includes:

- **Apply cold water to the burn area**; hose or garden spray or soaked sponges
- Avoid using wet towels or ice packs if possible (creates painful pressure on the wound)
- **Treat for shock**
- Keep the animal's **environmental temperature warm** to avoid hypothermia; use blanket and bubble wrap and avoid direct heat sources such as heat pads or heat lamps
- Clip and clean the area (this may not be possible in the unanaesthetised patient in which case leave until later)
- Apply **sterile waterproof nonstick dressing** to prevent loss of body fluids (a clean sheet of polythene applied directly over the area with cold wet flannel is a useful temporary measure)

CHEMICAL BURNS

- Restrain the animal's head or apply Elizabethan collar to **prevent it licking the chemical**
- **Wash the burned area** with copious volumes of water to remove the chemical from the skin
- For known **alkaline chemicals,** e.g. caustic soda, **apply an acid solution** of vinegar and water in equal quantities to neutralise the chemical
- For known **acidic chemicals** use an **alkali,** apply a concentrated solution of bicarbonate of soda

CHEST WALL INJURIES

Injury to the chest wall is painful and dyspnoea, pain, collapse and subcutaneous emphysema often result. Usually caused by road accidents, dog bites, gunshot or staking injuries. Clinical signs may not be seen, however, the main complication of chest wall injuries is collapse of the lung. Damage may result in an open pneumothorax, closed pneumothorax, haemothorax or diaphragmatic rupture.

- Administer **oxygen** (see Chapter 40)
- **Do not remove** any penetrating foreign bodies
- **Cover wounds** with 'Clingfilm' and Vaseline and dressings to prevent further pneumothorax

- **Strict rest** in quiet room/kennel to prevent stressing animal further
- Prepare for **radiography**

CONCUSSION

The signs of concussion vary, ranging from dazed and confused to unconscious. Other signs possible include shock, haemorrhage from ears, nose, mouth, unequally dilated pupils (anisocoria), nystagmus, slow shallow respiration, vomiting and paralysis.

- Maintain airway
- Monitor eye reflexes and degree of depression
- Treat shock (warm, fluids, etc.)

CONVULSIONS/SEIZURES/EPILEPTIFORM FITS

There are many causes that result in convulsions, including poisoning, tumours, heat stroke, epilepsy, brain trauma and metabolic disturbances (hypoglycaemia, hypocalcaemia). Most seizures result in unconsciousness and severe involuntary skeletal muscle contraction. Other signs include restlessness, salivation, pupil dilation and voiding urine and faeces.

- **Do not** restrain
- Move furniture away
- Keep in dark and quiet room
- Time length of seizure
- Obtain brief history from owner (possible exposure to poisons, lactating female, RTA)
- Remain calm, and advise owners to remain calm – although it looks frightening, in most cases, 'fits' are not fatal

CORNEAL DAMAGE

Ulcers, chemical splashes, paint and other toxins may cause surface damage to the corneal surface. Cat fight injuries, cactus spines and RTAs may cause penetrating wounds to the cornea. Surface damage may not be noticeable but there may be a blue/opaque patch on the eye. Penetrating injuries may result in the surface of the eye looking wrinkled.

EMERGENCY CARE

- **Flush eye** with sterile saline (tap water only when saline not available) to remove toxins, etc.
- Confine in **darkened room**
- **Do not disturb or remove any foreign bodies**
- Apply an **eye patch**/head bandage
- Apply an **Elizabethan collar**

DISLOCATIONS/LUXATIONS

A dislocation (or luxation) is the displacement of the articular surfaces of a joint. Commonly occurs in the carpal and tarsal joints, the hip joint and the elbow following RTAs. Clinical signs include unusual mobility, swelling around the joint, deformity, pain and limited movement of the joint.

- Do not reduce the dislocation
- Apply cold compress to the area to reduce swelling and ease pain
- Confine animal to prevent excessive movement
- Analgesics given by VETERINARY SURGEON

ELECTROCUTION

High voltage passes through the body, most commonly seen in young dogs chewing electric cables. The animal is usually found collapsed by the source of the problem. Clinical signs include thermal burns – necrosis of lips and tongue, dyspnoea, muscular contractions, body stiffness and unconsciousness

- **Switch off electricity supply** before touching the animal. If this cannot be done, move the animal away from the source with a **wooden pole**
- **Maintain airway**, administer oxygen and IPPV if necessary
- **Check heart rate** – give cardiac massage if necessary
- Treat thermal burns

EPISTAXIS

Caused by trauma to the head, tumours, foreign bodies and persistent sneezing. Clinical signs include haemorrhage, sneezing, open-mouth breathing, upper respiratory noise and dyspnoea.

- Cold compress applied to nose
- Constant observation
- Confine and calm patient
- Sedate if necessary

FISH-HOOKS

Fish-hooks have barbed ends and will cause pain and damage to the tissues if they are pulled out. The hook should be **pushed further** so that the **barb exits out through the skin**. The shaft of the hook can then be **cut with wire cutters**. The hook may then be pulled out. An antiseptic such **as povidone-iodine should be applied to the area. Sedation** of the patient may be required for removal.

FLAIL CHEST

Where multiple rib fractures result in a 'floating' section of the chest. This results in poor aeration of the underlying lung.

- The animal should be placed into **lateral recumbency** with the **affected side lowermost.** This will stabilise the flail from moving
- Give **oxygen**
- **IPPV** may be required to stabilise the respiratory pattern of the patient

FRACTURES

A fracture consists of a break in a bone. There are different types of fracture and they can be classified as:

Simple: The bone is broken cleanly, into two pieces

Compound: The fractured bones exit out of or can be seen through a skin wound

Complicated: Where other important structures have been damaged by the fractured bone (blood vessels, spinal cord, lungs, nerves, etc.)

Comminuted: Where there are many pieces of fractured bone at the fracture site

Multiple: Where the bone is fractured in more than one place or other bones are fractured

Avulsed: Where the fractured bone fragment is being pulled further away from its original position by a tendon

Over-riding: Each end of bone is pushed passed the other piece

Clinical signs seen with fractures include pain at the site of the fracture, swelling, loss of function, deformity of a part or limb, unnatural mobility and crepitus.

- **Confine** the animal to reduce movement of the fractured area.
- **Control haemorrhage** from wounds and compound fractures.
- **Treat shock.**
- **Clean wounds** – and compound fracture sites with warmed sterile saline and apply sterile dressing (refer to Wound section).
- **Support the fracture** – however, there is some dispute about whether or not to apply splints, Robert Jones bandages, etc. Each practice will have its own protocol. Applying such support to a conscious animal could cause more pain and injury than simply putting the animal in a cage to restrict movement. Most animals will not use a limb if it is fractured and will protect it naturally themselves, when lying down or moving. Splints, Robert Jones bandages or casts can be applied if necessary, when the animal is later anaesthetised for radiography.
- **Keep animal comfortable** – provide padding and warmth.

GASTRIC DILATATION/VOLVULUS (TORSION)

A condition most frequently seen in large, deep-chested breeds of dog shortly after they have eaten. The stomach fills up with gas and subsequently swells enormously. Sometimes the stomach then twists on itself and causes the torsion. In either case, this is a high priority **emergency situation**. The animal's circulatory system becomes severely compromised very quickly and the condition can be fatal if not treated immediately.

Clinical signs include: pain – animal in 'praying' position (orthopnoea), restlessness, abdominal swelling, laboured respiration and collapse

- **Relieve pressure in stomach** – pass stomach tube or if this is not possible, quickly aseptically prepare the skin to place an 18-gauge needle/intravenous catheter through the left abdominal wall at point of most distension and/or timpany
- **Administer fluid therapy** – compound sodium lactate at an infusion rate of 90 ml/kg/hour
- **Monitor and record vital signs**
- **Prepare for emergency surgery**

Note: Do not use acepromazine or other depressants, which will exacerbate hypovolaemia.

HAEMORRHAGE

Caused by numerous types of injuries, haemorrhage should be treated quickly – whether the blood loss is acute or chronic; both can result in hypovolaemia, shock and death.

- Apply **direct digital pressure** to the wound using clean hands or sterile swabs. Useful as a temporary measure in small wounds but should not be used in the presence of a penetrating foreign body in case object is pushed further into the wound.
- **Artery forceps** may be used **to close off specific arteries or veins** if it is possible to locate such bleeding points. Care must be taken not to damage too much surrounding tissue.
- **Gauze swabs or dressing pads** may be applied firmly to limb wounds and bandaged into place.
- **Doughnut ring bandages** may be used if there is a penetrating foreign body. If the blood soaks through the first layer apply more layers but do not disturb clot.
- For **internal bleeding** a crepe bandage **may be applied** to increase the back pressure.
- **Apply a tourniquet** to occlude an artery by pressing it against a bone to prevent further blood loss at a site lower down a limb or the tail.

There are three points in the dog and cat where tourniquets can be applied:

(1) **Brachial artery**: medial side of the humerus, distal third. Pressure applied prevents haemorrhage from below the elbow.

EMERGENCY CARE

(2) **Femoral artery**: medial aspect of the thigh, proximal third. Pressure applied will stop haemorrhage from below the stifle.
(3) **Coccygeal artery**: underside of the tail, pressure is applied at the root of the tail.

HOW TO APPLY A TOURNIQUET

- A tourniquet may be applied a few inches above the wound (between the heart and the wound)
- Adjust the tightness of the tourniquet to stop the blood flow
- A tourniquet must **not be left on more than 15 minutes** before it is moved or slackened to allow the tissues to recover
- Tourniquets should **only be used when other control methods have failed**

HEATSTROKE

Exposure to excessive heat especially in **brachycephalic** or **long-haired** dogs following **excessive exercise** or **high** environmental **temperatures** (e.g. confinement in a small space during hot weather).

The animal is usually distressed, panting excessively and restless. As the temperature increases the animal may collapse, salivating excessively. This then progresses into coma and death. Rectal temperatures of 41–43°C (105–110°F) indicate hyperthermia.

- Obtain core body temperature
- Maintain airway
- Provide oxygen if necessary
- Cool the animal down by one of these methods:
  - Hose with cold water (start with limbs and work up the body if necessary)
  - Cover the body in wet towels
  - Administer cold intravenous fluids
  - Apply isopropyl alcohol to pads on feet and ear flaps
  - Apply ice packs or bags of frozen vegetables (cover with thin cloth first to prevent ice burns)
- Check temperature every 3 minutes until within normal range

EMERGENCY CARE

- **Hospitalise** animal in a **well-ventilated room** and **confine** to prevent over-exertion. An oxygen cage cooled to 22°C (72°F) may be useful in smaller animals.

Note: it is important to remember that **cooling the animal too quickly may cause hypothermia** – small dogs and cats can become hypothermic in minutes following initial cooling, if possible obtain a **constant body temperature reading** during the cooling process.

HYPOCALCAEMIA (ECLAMPSIA, LACTATION TETANY)

Usually seen in lactating bitches with large litters, 2–5 weeks after parturition. The milk demand by the offspring causes huge drains on the dam's calcium levels. If the diet does not provide enough calcium the dam becomes hypocalcaemic (low blood calcium levels).

Signs include (in increasing severity), restlessness, panting, tachypnoea, muscular spasms, collapse, hyperaesthesia, unconsciousness and latterly, death.

- Veterinary surgeon to **administer 10% calcium solution intravenously**. Calcium borogluconate (0.5–1.5 ml/kg of 10% solution over 20–30 minutes).
- **Constantly observe and monitor** dam during administration (hypotension may develop after i/v administration).
- **Remove offspring** and use an alternative feeding method for them.

HYPOGLYCAEMIA

May occur in the diabetic patient when either too much insulin has been given or if the animal has not eaten in the period after administration of insulin or if the animal has over-exercised. Blood glucose levels become dramatically reduced and cause signs such as lethargy, apparent blindness, ataxia, collapse, convulsions, coma and death.

- Give oral glucose solution, chocolate, honey, glucose (rub onto gums if the animal is unconscious)
- Veterinary surgeon to administer glucose by intravenous injection (1–5 ml 50% dextrose slowly over 10 minutes, ideally via a jugular catheter as 10–50% solutions are irritant)

- Constantly observe and monitor patient during administration

HYPOTHERMIA

Causes include cold environmental conditions, anaesthesia, inactivity, malnutrition and hypothyroidism.

- **Administer warmed intravenous fluids** – heat the bag and place as much as possible of the administration set through a container of warmed water
- Veterinary surgeon to administer warmed intraperitoneal fluids (20 ml/kg repeated at 30 minute intervals until body temperature is normal)
- **Increase ambient room temperature** or place small animals into heated oxygen cage
- Place animal on **heat pads, water bed, hot water bottles** (ensure these are covered to prevent thermal burns)
- Cover the animal in **space blanket or bubble wrap**
- Monitor core temperature frequently to prevent hyperthermia
- Do not warm too quickly
- Auscultate **heart** for arrhythmias

Note: hypothermia is frequently responsible for slow anaesthetic recoveries. It is your responsibility to obtain a core body temperature from *all* animals following anaesthesia and act appropriately.

Plastic bags filled with corn heated in a microwave make useful and inexpensive 'heat pads', which will stay warm for long periods. Disposable gloves filled with hot water can be used as hot water bottles, as can empty plastic drink bottles. Always cover these with a towel or blanket to make sure they don't burn the animal.

INSECT STINGS

The mouth and front paws are the most common areas affected by wasp and bee stings. Stings may cause excessive swelling, discomfort and in some cases severe allergic reaction resulting in collapse. If the animal has been stung in the back of the throat, the swelling may be enough to cause serious airway obstruction.

- Treat **shock**
- **Provide oxygen** therapy if animal is dyspnoeic
- **Veterinary surgeon to give corticosteroids** intravenously
- **Scrape** the 'sting' away if has not been embedded into skin or
- **Pull sting out using forceps** if it is already embedded into the skin – as close to the skin surface as possible to avoid bursting the poison sacs
- If the owners know what stung the animal:
  - Use **bicarbonate** (1 tsp. bicarbonate: 250 ml water) to bathe and neutralise the area for **bee stings**
  - Use **vinegar** (50:50 with water) for **wasp** stings to bathe the area

PARAPHIMOSIS

Constriction of the prepuce around an engorged penis so that the penis cannot be retracted back into the prepuce can occur in the dog. If neglected, gangrene of the tip of the penis may result. Clinically, the penis is very dry, swollen and reddened.

- Apply a cold compress
- Apply KY gel or liquid paraffin to tip of penis to lubricate tissues
- Reduce the paraphimosis if possible. If not possible, keep the penis moist until surgical repair is carried out

POISONING

It is important that you have a basic understanding of the first aid treatment of any animal that has been poisoned and so you need to know a lot of background knowledge.

Poisons enter the animal's body by:

- Ingestion (eating)
- Inhalation (inhaling noxious fumes)
- Absorption (absorption through paws, eyes, mucous membranes, etc.)

You must obtain a history from the owner to aid diagnosis (many of the clinical signs seen in poisoning cases can be confused with other illnesses and disorders, e.g. epilepsy, heatstroke, severe gastro-enteritis.).

IDENTIFY THE TYPE OF POISON

- Obtain a case history from owner, asking questions like:
  - Did you see the animal eat the poison? If so, bring sample to surgery
  - What poisons are at home? Give suggestions, often people don't even know that certain substances are poisonous
  - How long ago was it eaten?
  - Has the animal been sick?
- Examine the animal – record temperature, pulse and respiration and act on these if abnormal
- Obtain samples of voided body fluids (vomit, blood, urine, faeces)

PREVENT FURTHER ABSORPTION OF THE POISON

- **Induce emesis** if within 4 hours of ingestion **only** if poison is **noncorrosive**
- **Administer gastric lavage**
- **Administer oxygen** or plenty of fresh air if the poison was inhaled
- **Flush area** with copious amounts of **water** if poison was absorbed through skin

REMOVE THE POISON

Induce emesis if ingested within the last hour: do not induce emesis if corrosive substance ingested (e.g. disinfectants – phenols, QACs, petroleum products).

Administer one of the following to induce emesis:

- Apomorphine 0.04 mg/kg I/V or 0.08 mg/kg I/M (veterinary surgeon to give).
- Xylazine ('Rompun') 0.5 mg/kg I/V (veterinary surgeon to give). Sedation may add to complications.
- Washing soda crystal, walnut-sized (may be corrosive!).
- Salt water (2 tsp. in cup of warm water). May cause hypernatraemia.
- Mustard and water (2 tsp. in a cup of warm water).

Gastric lavage is useful if carried out within 4 hours of ingestion

- Water
- Saline
- Fullers earth or charcoal added to mixture to absorb toxins

Place a stomach tube and holding the tube up high, pour in 5–10 ml/kg of **warmed** water or saline. Rotate the animal to mix the fluid in the stomach. Lower the tube into a bucket and allow fluid to be siphoned off. Repeat at least ten times. Add fullers earth (BCK) or charcoal during last few flushes to absorb any remaining poison.

- BCK granules (1–3 tbsp. mixed into paste with water)
- Charcoal (1 g/kg) mixed with water)

Use of cathartics. (A cathartic is a substance that encourages the passage of the ingestate through the gastrointestinal tract. In other words, it helps to speed up the elimination of the poison through and out of the body.)

- 40% sodium sulphate solution may be used at a dose rate of 1 g/kg

Use of demulcents. (A demulcent coats the alimentary lining with a soothing substance to protect and relieve the mucosal surface along the alimentary tract. Especially useful when a corrosive has been ingested.)

- One beaten raw egg, milk, one teaspoon sugar by mouth

TREAT CLINICAL SIGNS AND KEEP ANIMAL COMFORTABLE

- Treat shock, seizures, dyspnoea, hypothermia and hyperthermia.
- Give antidote.
- Veterinary surgeon to give antidote if poison and its antidote known, e.g. vitamin K, (Konakion™) for warfarin (rat bait) poisoning.

SET UP INTRAVENOUS FLUIDS

Most poisons are eventually metabolised by the liver and then excreted through the kidneys. Give I/V fluids to speed up removal of the poison out of the body and to help dilute the toxin to reduce damage on the cells of the kidney. The veterinary surgeon may administer or add a diuretic to the fluid to increase the rate of excretion.

Notes: It is important that you do not get involved in *any* discussion with owners about malicious poisonings. Never agree with, suggest or provoke conversation about this subject – remain impartial at all times.

Have the telephone number of the Veterinary Poisons Information Service (VPIS) to hand always. They provide 24-hour information service (for the UK) about poisons and the methods of treatment. The VN is only allowed to contact the VPIS with the consent of the VS! There is a charge for this service. The number is: **020 7635 9195** or **0113 245 0530**.

PROLAPSED EYEBALL

Injury to the orbital area (RTAs, fights, etc.) can result in the eye prolapsing. This is more likely to occur in brachycephalic breeds with a shallow orbit and protuberant eyes. The eyeball sits out from the rest of the face, is usually inflamed and very dry. It is important to replace the eye as quickly as possible before other damage occurs to the unprotected eyeball, and the cornea ulcerates and the optic nerve becomes permanently damaged.

- **Lubricate the eye** and keep it moist using artificial tears or liquid paraffin
- **Replace eyeball by pulling eyelids over the eye** – this should only be carried out by qualified personnel
- **Do not push the eye** back in to the socket, if the method above does not work, keep the eyeball lubricated using saline (advise owners to use contact lens solution or 1/2 tsp. salt:1 litre cool, boiled water)
- Apply **Elizabethan collar**
- **Treat shock**

PROLAPSED RECTUM

Sever tenesmus as a result of either diarrhoea or constipation can cause the rectum to protrude through the anal sphincter. Most frequently seen in young puppies or kittens (and hamsters!). The length of prolapse varies, but appears as a pink/

EMERGENCY CARE

red oedematous, tubular structure – like a sausage, from the anus. If left, the rectum dries out and may ulcerate.

- **Moisten and lubricate** the prolapsed tissue using warm saline to clean first and then liquid paraffin to lubricate tissues
- **Replace prolapse** by gently pinching the end of the prolapse with the finger and thumb to encourage the tip of the prolapse to turn back in on itself
- If unsuccessful, apply **Elizabethan collar**
- **Prevent further straining,** by spraying prolapse with local analgesic agent (lignocaine) until surgical correction can be carried out

RUPTURED DIAPHRAGM

Usually caused by RTAs or direct trauma, the diaphragm tears and allows the abdominal organs to pass through into the thoracic cavity, which, in turn, causes the lungs to collapse. Dyspnoea in varying degrees of severity may result. These animals often take an unusual positional stance (orthopnoea).

- Oxygen therapy
- Cage rest in stress-free environment (away from barking dogs, etc.)
- Place animal on a sloped surface, so that head is higher than hindquarters. This encourages the abdominal organs to fall back into the abdomen and reduces pressure on the lungs and heart.
- Monitor patient constantly until surgery

SHOCK

Shock occurs in nearly **all accident and trauma victims**. You must never underestimate the effects of even minor accidents on the cardiovascular system. Your role in providing any first aid treatment for animals is mainly concerned with shock control and you must be fully familiar with the clinical signs of shock. **Remember, do not wait** until an animal is showing signs of shock, and instead **prevent shock occurring in the first place.** This means, that you should **initiate basic shock control for *all* accident victims** unless otherwise instructed by a qualified member of staff.

The clinical signs of shock become more pronounced the more severe the shock is, but include in increasing severity:

- Pale, clammy mucous membranes
- Slow capillary refill time (>2 seconds)
- Tachypnoea
- Tachycardia
- Rapid but feeble weak pulse (you may not be able to palpate a peripheral pulse)
- Cold extremities
- Hypothermia
- Depression, lethargy and collapse

TREATMENT INCLUDES

- **Correct or remove** the cause of shock, e.g. control haemorrhage (refer to specific first aid treatments as listed).
- **Provide warmth,** and prevent further heat loss – blankets, space blankets, etc.
- **Prepare warmed intravenous fluids.**
- **Observe constantly.**
- **Monitor and record vital signs** – it is essential that you record your findings of vital signs so that trends can be determined – either improvements in the patient's condition or deterioration. Make notes on the general demeanour of the animal.
- Provide **comfort and sympathetic nursing** – these animals are often confused, stressed and disorientated. Handle them gently and stoke and encourage them during the recovery period.

SPINAL INJURY

Usually as a result of RTA or disc protrusion following chronic disease. Rabbits can sustain spinal fractures if restrained improperly. These patients are usually in intense pain, are unable to move or get up and cry out in pain if moved. Animals that are not paraplegic or quadriplegic often take up a strange positional stance and are ataxic.

- **Do not move** unless necessary
- **Carry on rigid board**
- **Treat shock** and keep warm

WOUNDS

There are many classifications of wounds depending on the area damaged and the extent of the damage. First aid treatment of wounds obviously depends on these factors but generally, first aid care consists of:

CLOSED WOUNDS – CONTUSIONS AND HAEMATOMA

- **Ice packs** should be applied in the first instance to reduce the incidence of swelling.
- **Pressure bandages** can be applied to control haemorrhage and reduce swelling but should only be left on for up to 12 hours.
- In the later stages, **hot compresses** may help to reduce the pain.

OPEN WOUNDS – LACERATIONS, PUNCTURES, PENETRATING WOUNDS AND ABRASIONS

- **Remove the cause of the wound** if still in place (e.g. fishhook)
- **Control haemorrhage** if necessary
- **Control shock**, keep animal warm
- If possible, **clip around the wounds** to remove large amounts of fur (this may stress animal so leave until anaesthetised)
- **Clean wound** using copious amounts of **sterile saline** or water and very dilute solution of iodine if saline not available (warm the fluids to body temperature)
- **Cover the wound** with appropriate sterile dressing and bandage appropriately
- Apply **Elizabethan collar** to prevent self-trauma

FURTHER READING

Bistner, S.I. & Ford, R.B. (1995) *Handbook of Veterinary Procedures and Emergency Treatment,* 6th edn. WB Saunders Company, London.

APPENDIX 1

CARE PLANS FOR SURGICAL AND MEDICAL CONDITIONS

Animals with different conditions and diseases have many different nursing care requirements and it is important that you are aware of each patient's specific needs and how to go about caring for them during hospitalisation. Close observational skills, being aware of potential problems and being able to provide a high level of nursing care will help to ensure patient comfort and speed up rehabilitation, thus reducing hospitalisation stays.

As described in Chapters 1 and 3, thorough daily assessment and measurement of vital signs is essential. A temperature, pulse and respiratory measurement should be obtained *at least* once a day for *every* hospitalised patient. In addition to this, the following care plans are designed to give a quick point of reference for the additional care required for some of the common surgical and medical conditions. It should be remembered however, that each patient's needs are unique and you must discuss appropriate care plans for every hospitalised animal with the veterinary surgeon in charge.

CARE PLANS FOR GENERAL CONDITIONS

BANDAGES

An animal is likely to interfere with a bandage if it has become uncomfortable or too tight. In the event of patient interference, always check the bandage first. As a guide, you should just be able to insert a finger into the proximal and distal ends of the bandage. Boredom is another cause of interference so toys and time spent grooming the patient can be help to remedy the problem.

- Check the bandage frequently and change it if it becomes soiled, wet or loose.

- Ensure that limb bandages are applied to the entire limb; partly covering a limb may cause swelling distal to the bandage.
- If the toes are exposed, assess to ensure adequate blood flow to the area.
- Apply Elizabethan collar if necessary to prevent interference.
- When taking the animal outside, cover the lower part of the bandage with a protective covering. An empty drip bag with the end cut off provides a sturdy cover, which can be reused. Always remove the bag as soon as the patient is returned to the kennel.
- Remove pressure bandages after 12 hours of application.

FEEDING TUBES

More detail regarding placement and care of feeding tubes has been given in Chapter 4. In addition to monitoring vital signs, it is beneficial to palpate the lymph nodes nearest the tube insertion for evidence of enlargement, indicating infection at the tube site.

Where pharyngostomy or gastrotomy tubes have been placed:

- Cover the tube insertion area with povidone-iodine ointment and a sterile keyhole dressing. See Fig. A1.1.
- Cover entire area with padding and bandage to prevent the tube dangling or becoming dislodged. Stockinet bandage is particularly useful as a final layer over the padding.
- Clean the incision site daily with antiseptic soap and water.
- Flush the tube with 5 ml of water before and after feeding to prevent tube blockage.
- Always ensure that the end of the tube is plugged before and after feeding (an intravenous needle cap may be used if a spigot is unavailable).
- Prevent patient interference with an Elizabethan collar.
- Observe the patient for evidence of vomiting, regurgitation or bloating.
- Check for diarrhoea. If present, you may need to dilute feeding solution.
- Monitor body weight daily.
- In the event of tube displacement or aspiration of food, stop feeding and remove the tube.

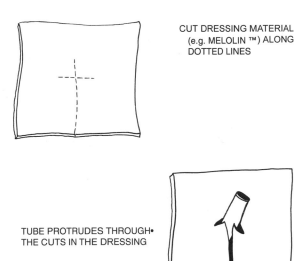

CUT DRESSING MATERIAL
(e.g. MELOLIN ™) ALONG
DOTTED LINES

TUBE PROTRUDES THROUGH•
THE CUTS IN THE DRESSING

Fig. A1.1   Keyhole dressing.

Where a nasogastric tube has been placed:

- Ensure that the tube is still secured to the animal's facial skin.
- Check the tube frequently to ensure that the distal end has not become displaced (observe for coughing).
- Ensure feeding solution is sufficiently dilute and liquid to pass through the narrow bore of the tube.
- Test the tube position before each feed by syringing 1–2 ml of sterile saline (saline will be absorbed quickly if inserted into the trachea).

INTRAVENOUS CATHETERS

The main nursing consideration for patients with an intravenous catheter is to maintain a patent line and prevent sepsis. Complications are more likely the longer the catheter is left in place and so strict aseptic techniques should be applied to prevent nosocomial infection.

- Wash hands before handling the catheter and associated connectors or fluid lines.
- Examine catheter site for signs of infection (erythema, swelling).
- Palpate lymph nodes above and around catheter site each day during placement.

- Obtain core body temperature twice daily to detect pyrexia.
- Wipe catheter junctions and bungs with 70% isopropyl alcohol before handling or injecting any drugs.
- Flush the catheter 2–4 times a day with heparinised saline to prevent coagulation and thrombus formation.
- Administer drugs slowly.
- Clamp off the proximal line on any administration lines to ensure that the drug enters the patient and not the fluid bag.
- Apply a topical antibiotic preparation or povidone-iodine over catheter entry site to reduce risk of catheter-related sepsis.
- Bandage entire catheter in place to help prevent contamination and patient interference.
- Use a splint or bandage to extend the limb to prevent kinking of the catheter.
- Change bandage if it becomes soiled.
- Remove the catheter as soon as it is no longer required.
- Change catheter site every 3 days (7 days for jugular catheters).
- Take care when removing the bandage and catheter. Cut bandages on the opposite aspect of the limb from the catheter to prevent cutting through the catheter needle.

RECUMBENCY

Causes of recumbency range from unconsciousness and debilitation to severe spinal trauma. Recumbent patients are often hospitalised for long periods and easily become bored or stressed. They require the intensive nursing techniques as described below as well the additional time spent keeping them company and interested. It may be beneficial to call owners in to sit with the animal for short periods each day to help with this aspect of the rehabilitation of these animals.

- Provide a kennel large enough for the patient to lie in lateral recumbency but not so large that the animal is able to drag itself around and cause distress.
- If possible, place the patient in an area of activity to help provide stimulation and relieve boredom.

- Ensure soft, warm, comfortable bedding with lots of padding. Use a foam mattress and thick bedding, e.g. Vetbed and an incontinence pad if necessary.
- Recumbent animals become cold easily so provide additional heating if necessary. Take care not to burn the animal, who cannot move away from the heat source.
- Keep food and water within reach and hand feed if necessary.
- Feed highly palatable, concentrated and easily digestible food (less faeces!) and consider reducing quantity of food because of the lack of exercise.
- Increase the fibre content of food if the patient becomes constipated.
- Take outside if appropriate, using a towel sling.
- Clean and groom the patient daily. Patients may be unable to do this for themselves and it will help reduce boredom.
- Apply talcum powder on areas where skin may rub such as the inguinal region.
- Massage limbs to aid circulation.
- Clean any decubital ulcers with mild antiseptic solution, dry thoroughly and apply white soft paraffin followed by a 'doughnut' dressing.
- Turn patient 3–4 hourly.
- Perform coupage 3–4 times daily (see Chapter 7) to aid removal of secretions by coughing.
- Encourage sternal recumbency using sandbags, foam wedges or rolled up bedding.
- Prevent urine/faecal scalds by thoroughly cleaning the patient and applying white soft paraffin around the perianal area. Clipping the hair around the perianal area will aid cleaning especially in long-haired breeds.
- Check bladder frequently to ensure it does not become overdistended. Manually express the bladder if instructed to do so by the veterinary surgeon.

TECHNIQUE FOR MANUALLY EXPRESSING THE BLADDER

By squeezing the bladder gently so that pressure increases, the urinary sphincter is opened and urine should flow out.

- Place a hand on either side of the caudal abdomen over the bladder.

APPENDICES

- When you can feel the bladder, apply gentle continuous pressure.
- Diazepam and phenoxybenzamine (Dibenylin) may be administered according to the veterinary surgeon's instructions to help relax the urinary sphincter. You can then manually express 20–30 minutes later.

TRACHEOTOMY TUBES

Animals with tracheotomies require intensive monitoring and a high level of care. Tube hygiene is essential and in the initial stages, the tube may need to be cleaned as often as every 15–30 minutes. The newer plastic tubes with a removable inner tube are preferable to the metal tubes as they are better tolerated by the patient and enable easier and more thorough cleaning of the tube.

- Clean tracheotomy wound at least daily with antiseptic solution, removing accumulated exudate, and apply povidone-iodine ointment to help protect the skin wound.
- Cover the tube incision site with a keyhole dressing around the tracheotomy tube.
- Observe the animal closely to ensure the tube does not become occluded with bandaging materials, skin folds or bedding. (Do not use 'Vetbed' type bedding material, which may clog the tube entrance.)
- Ensure the tube is securely attached to the patient and tape in position to prevent dislodgement.
- Instil 1–5 ml of sterile saline down the tube into the trachea every 1–2 hours. This will help to moisturise the trachea, humidify the inspired air and loosen mucous debris.
- Aspirate tracheal secretions by suction using a sterile urethral dog catheter and syringe. Animals with tracheotomies are not able to cough to remove any tracheal secretions.
- Clean the tube frequently. Ideally use a cannulated tube so that the inner tube can be removed for cleaning.
- Prevent self-trauma but use Elizabethan collars with extreme care as they may interfere with the tracheotomy site. Bandage feet if necessary.

URINARY CATHETERS

Studies have shown that after 4 days of closed urine collection, most catheterised patients develop urinary tract infections (UTI) despite being given antibiotic therapy. It is recommended therefore that an indwelling urinary catheter should not be left in place for more than 24 hours and that a closed collection system is used to help prevent UTI. You must observe the patient closely for development of pyrexia, discomfort, pyuria and other signs of UTI.

- Wash hands and wear disposable gloves (for your own safety precautions) before handling and checking catheter and lines
- Ensure that the urine drainage bag is lower than the level of patient's bladder to prevent urine flow back
- Check lines and catheter to ensure they do not become kinked or blocked
- Prevent self-trauma by applying Elizabethan collar
- Apply an antibacterial ointment to the urethral orifice

WOUND DRAINS

Potential complications include wound breakdown, ascending infection, blockage and local tissue irritation. You must carry out effective hygiene procedures during the nursing of these patients and observe the animal closely for evidence of infection.

- Ensure that the drain is sutured securely to the skin
- Clean the drain entry and exit site and surrounding skin daily with an antiseptic solution
- Cover the drain entry sites with sterile keyhole dressings
- Apply white soft paraffin around and below the drain exit site to prevent skin excoriation
- Bandage area with highly absorbent dressing such as cotton wool to soak up secretions and secure in place using Stockinet-type bandage
- Prevent self-trauma by applying an Elizabethan collar

GERIATRICS

Geriatric patients admitted to the surgery require particular attention in order to try to maintain their normal routine. You should obtain information from the owner regarding their normal lifestyle and treatment at home. Older animals frequently suffer from other diseases and you should implement appropriate nursing care for each condition. In addition, ensure that any existing medication plans are continued, checking first that they are not contra-indicated with any new treatment being prescribed.

- Ensure that water is available ad lib and monitor and record intake quantities
- Feed a high quality protein to help reduce muscle mass loss, but not high levels of protein in cases where there is existing kidney disease
- Give small, frequent highly palatable meals rather than overloading digestive system and organs with one or two large feed volumes per day
- If necessary, reduce the quantity being given to help reduce obesity
- Provide soft, warm, comfortable, easily washable bedding for comfort and to help prevent decubitus ulcers over bony prominences.
- Additional heating may be required due to poor circulation
- Keep away from draughts
- Ensure frequent but short trips outside help to reduce incontinence problems and reduce stiffness
- Groom the patient daily as geriatric patients are less likely to clean themselves
- Handle gently and take care as older animals are more likely to become irritable and snap at handlers

NEONATES

If the dam dies, loses her milk supply or becomes hypocalcaemic the neonates will have to be hand-reared. If the young have not already received some colostrum, try to milk some from the mammary glands of the dam (provided it is not contaminated with drugs or toxins) and give to the young in one of their first feeds. Orphaned offspring are at a higher risk of getting infections because they have often not received any colostrum and therefore do not have any maternal antibodies. Thorough hygiene is essential.

- Always wash your hands before handling.
- Place orphans into an incubator if available or use infrared lamp, hot water bottles or heated corn pad. Take care not to

cause burns. Remember also, not to let the temperature drop at night time. The ambient temperature should be 24–27°C (75–80°F) for the first 10 days and reducing gradually to room temperature by week four.

- Always sterilise feeding equipment before each use.
- Use commercial milk substitute. Cow's milk and goat's milk are not suitable. Examples of milk substitutes include Lactol, Pedigree Instant Milk Substitute, Welpi, Cimicat and Whiskas Instant Milk Substitute.
- Use Catac or Hagan pet feeding bottle (use in preference to stomach tube, which does not satisfy their natural sucking reflex).
- Calculate required amount according to manufacturer's instructions.
- Sterilise feeding equipment in Milton sterilising fluid.
- Warm food to body temperature before feeding (39°C).
- Feed every 2–4 hours throughout the day and night for the first few days then reduce to every 4 hours.
- Hold the neonate in sternal recumbency during feeding to encourage the natural paddling movement of limbs.
- After feeding, stimulate the young to pass urine and faeces by rubbing their abdomen and peri-anal region with a piece of warm, damp cotton wool until they void both (record all motions – bottle-fed young are prone to constipation).
- Clean the animal using warm, damp cotton wool – wipe around their mouth and nose to remove dried milk and clean around the rest of the body.
- Some humidity is important and can be provided by placing a piece of damp towelling near their box.

CARE PLANS FOR PATIENTS WITH MEDICAL CONDITIONS

Patients admitted to the hospital for a medical work up will frequently undergo many diagnostic tests before a therapeutic plan is worked out specifically for them. You may be responsible for obtaining and processing laboratory samples (Section 6) and taking radiographs (Chapter 27) as well as other diagnostic tools.

Once a diagnosis has been established, the nursing care should be tailored to meet the individual requirements of the patient. The following care plans highlight nursing considerations for some of the common medical conditions seen in hospitalised patients. As previously mentioned, it is especially imperative that vital signs are monitored frequently and the patient clinically assessed so that changes and deterioration can be picked up as quickly as possible.

BLOOD TRANSFUSIONS

Specific information regarding the method and rates of administration for blood transfusion has been given in Chapter 41. In addition you must constantly monitor the patient during and following transfusion.

- Obtain and record vital signs every 5 minutes
- Pay particular attention to any changes in mucous membrane colour, capillary refill time, pulse quality and core temperature
- Observe for evidence of transfusion reaction (refer to Chapter 41)
- Stop transfusion and seek veterinary advice if you suspect a transfusion reaction
- Be prepared to set up oxygen and fluid therapy if necessary
- Ensure transfusion is being given at the prescribed rate
- Wash hands before handling administration set and wear sterile gloves when handling catheter
- Obtain a PCV every 2–4 hours following transfusion

CHEMOTHERAPY

Cancer patients require a high level of nursing attention and skill. These animals are often hospitalised for long periods and easily become depressed and anorexic. Cancer patients have impaired immune function and are therefore more susceptible to infection so good hygiene is essential.

The drugs used for chemotherapy are highly cytotoxic. Most chemotherapy agents are cytotoxic, mutogenic and teratogenic and present a real danger to operators. You must exercise extreme care at all times when they are used and during the nursing of recipient patients.

- Wear two pairs of gloves at all times when handling cytotoxic drugs and during any time when dealing with the animal

- Avoid cutting or breaking tablets if possible and wear a mask if this must be done
- Wear disposable plastic aprons
- Reconstitute cytotoxic drugs in a plastic tray (e.g. cat litter tray) to contain any spillages and ease cleaning
- Reconstitute cytotoxic drugs in a well-ventilated room but ensure doors and windows are closed to prevent draughts
- Cover all cuts and scratches
- Wear protective goggles
- Wear a good quality surgical face mask if reconstituting cytotoxic powders
- Use insulin syringes or luer-locking syringes and giving sets to prevent accidental leakage of cytotoxic drugs
- Wrap a sterile gauze pad around the top of any glass vials when opening them to prevent spillage
- Cap all needles before expelling air from the syringe or expel into the vial or ampoule
- Wrap sterile gauze pad around the needle when removing it from an injection port to help prevent needle-stick injury
- Use pill cutter when cutting cytotoxic drugs. Label cutter and only ever use with cytotoxic drugs
- Clearly label all drip bags containing cytotoxic agents

Administration of cytotoxic drugs

- Wear protective clothing (two pairs of gloves, apron, goggles)
- Prepare all necessary equipment for aseptic administration of drugs
- Check dosage
- Always administer chemotherapy drugs via an intravenous catheter to avoid accidental perivascular injection
- Inspect the infusion line and check the patency of the route with a large volume of 0.9% normal saline
- Ensure the correct administration rate
- Constantly supervise the patient and frequently check the vein for swelling and/or leakage at the site
- Stop infusion if animal appears to experience pain at injection site
- If the patient shows any evidence of interfering with the catheter or infusion line, apply an Elizabethan collar
- Flush infusion lines and catheters with 0.9% saline between drugs and/or after administration

Patient management

- Put up warning signs on kennels and any equipment used. 'Toxic tape' is useful to label kennels, drip bags and clinical waste bags.
- Wash hands frequently.
- Wear disposable protective gloves and aprons when cleaning out kennel and handling the patient's excreta (wear disposable shoe covers if there is a danger of urine contaminating shoes).
- Wear protective clothing when handling the animal and cleaning out the kennel.
- Dispose of all clinical waste including kennel excreta and newspaper, infusion lines, syringes, swabs, etc. into 'high-risk' clinical waste sacks. Double bag all waste and dispose in the normal way for incineration.
- Double bag all bedding and label with 'cytotoxic contamination wear gloves to handle'. Machine wash as normal.
- Take patient to a designated outdoor run to urinate. Due to the high rate of fluid administration during the therapy, patients will need to urinate more frequently.
- Rinse run with copious amounts of water after each use.
- Wear protective overshoes or specially designated Wellington boots.

DIABETES

Hospitalised patients with diabetes are likely to be either unstabilised and admitted for monitoring, or stabilised patients coming in for surgery. You must be able to recognise signs of hypoglycaemia (shivering, weakness, tachycardia, and seizures) and the signs of hyperglycaemia (diabetic coma).

- Closely observe clinical signs and maintain accurate and thorough records regarding appetite.
- Monitor and maintain accurate and thorough records of blood glucose testing and administration of insulin.
- Adhere to a strict routine for feeding time and quantity, time of insulin administration and exercise.
- Encourage the patient to eat. In the event of inappetance an animal is more unlikely to eat a prescription diet but it is important to get them eating something so try any palatable food.

- Diabetic animals undergoing anaesthesia are starved as usual but given half their usual dose of insulin on the morning of the procedure. Blood glucose should then be tested.
- If blood glucose levels are low then a glucose saline infusion may be administered during anaesthesia and blood glucose levels retested following surgery.
- During stabilisation, blood glucose should be monitored every 4 hours.
- When administering insulin, gently agitate the insulin bottle before withdrawing the insulin and do not wipe the rubber stopper with isopropyl alcohol.

DIARRHOEA

There are many causes of diarrhoea. Diarrhoea may be secondary to some other organ dysfunction such as renal failure or hepatic disease and so further nursing skills must be initiated. Other causes of diarrhoea are infectious and/or zoonotic and until a diagnosis is established it is advisable to barrier nurse the patient. Complications include dehydration and weight loss.

- Withhold food for 24 hours
- Offer small amounts of oral electrolyte solution or water and monitor fluid intake
- Assess hydration status frequently for early detection of dehydration
- Manage fluid therapy, check patency of lines and rate of administration
- Record frequency, consistency and colour of diarrhoea
- Ensure the patient and kennel are kept clean
- Take particular care with your own personal hygiene precautions

HEART DISEASE

Animals with acute cardiac problems require close observation and as little handling and stress as is possible in the hospital environment. You should also remember that some older patients will have cardiac disease even though they have been admitted for another reason.

APPENDICES

- Do not stress the animal, handle as little as possible and keep the animal in a quiet area preferably away from other animals. A towel partially covering the kennel door may be of benefit.
- Monitor the patient as frequently as advised by the veterinary surgeon. It will help to detect early any deterioration in the condition.
- Restrict exercise and cage rest. Provide short trips outside to urinate especially if diuretics are being administered.
- Keep the patient warm as peripheral circulation may be compromised.
- Prepare and provide oxygen therapy if the patient becomes cyanotic or dyspnoeic.
- Ensure that the correct drug doses and administration times are applied.
- Provide an appropriate diet such as low sodium and restrict calories if the patient is obese.
- Be confident in setting up and using cardiac monitoring equipment such as electrocardiograms, pulse oximeters and blood pressure monitors.

LIVER DISEASE

Hepatitis or inflammation of the liver is used to describe many diseases of the liver such as drug toxicity, viruses, infectious disease and neoplasia. Clinical signs (except jaundice and ascites) are wide-ranging and vague and may not be present until 80% or more of hepatic tissue is damaged.

Removal of the causal agent may not be possible, so the treatment and care plan may be supportive and symptomatic.

- Provide a stress-free environment and cage rest the patient to minimise discomfort.
- Handle the patient carefully and gently, patients with liver disease often have severe abdominal pain.
- Assist feed the patient if necessary. Many patients with hepatic disease become inappetent and anorexic.
- Provide a diet high in calories, but try to avoid a high protein diet, as metabolism may be impaired. Fat content should be minimised.
- Supplement vitamins (such as vitamins B, C and K) as prescribed by the veterinary surgeon.

APPENDICES

- If diuretics are being administered, provide adequate opportunities to urinate.
- Observe for clotting disorders, seizure activity, jaundice and ascites.

PANCREATITIS

Causes of pancreatitis include amongst others, infection, duct obstruction, trauma, drugs and hypercalcaemia. Acute pancreatitis is a life-threatening condition and permanent impairment of endocrine and / or exocrine function can occur as a result.

Clinical signs include vomiting, anorexia, diarrhoea and depression. Refer to the appropriate care plan in this chapter for details of specific nursing protocols. The aim of the care plan is to alleviate the clinical signs and provide supportive therapy whilst enabling the pancreas to return (as much as possible) to its normal function.

- Withhold food and water for 3–4 days to avoid stimulation of the pancreatic enzymes and allow the pancreas to rest.
- Maintain intravenous fluid therapy treatment at rates to replace fluid deficits and maintain hydration during the starvation period.
- Administer analgesia as prescribed by the veterinary surgeon to relieve abdominal pain. These patients will often demonstrate abdominal pain by adopting the 'prayer' position.
- When there has been no episode of vomiting for 1 or 2 days, small amounts of water can be introduced.
- If water is tolerated, small amounts of food may be given. A high carbohydrate (rice, pasta, potatoes), low protein and low fat diet should be given to help prevent a relapse. On the first day give only one-third of the usual calorific requirements, increasing to two-thirds on day two and full amount by day three.
- Monitor blood and urine glucose for the presence of diabetes mellitus.
- Monitor patient for development of disseminated intravascular coagulation (DIC), e.g. platelet counts and prothrombin time.

RENAL DISEASE

Signs of renal disease occur when there is loss of function of more than 75% of the nephrons and renal failure has occurred. The kidneys are no longer able to maintain the regulatory, excretory and endocrine functions and as a result fluid, electrolyte and acid-base imbalances occur. Treatment plans for *chronic* and *acute* renal failure vary slightly, but both include elimination of the underlying cause (if possible) and supporting the patient until renal function has been restored.

- Provide a quiet, stress-free and warm environment for the patient.
- Administer fluid therapy at prescribed rates to replace fluid losses and maintain hydration.
- It is essential to monitor urine output as this provides one of the most important indicators of renal function in the severely compromised patient. In the event of anuria, fluid therapy may be discontinued.
- Observe nursing care plan for those patients with indwelling urinary catheters and urine collection systems. (Refer to General Care Plans earlier in this chapter.)
- Feed little and often and give a diet of reduced protein of high biological value to minimise metabolic wastes and keep blood urea nitrogen levels as near to normal as possible.
- Provide unlimited access to water.
- Assist feed if the patient is anorexic.
- Obtain blood samples for urea nitrogen, creatinine and potassium concentration as requested by the veterinary surgeon.
- Provide opportunities for the patient to urinate frequently; a clean litter tray for cats and frequent trips outside for dogs.

RESPIRATORY COMPROMISE

Caring for animals with respiratory compromise can range from those with a nasal discharge to acute respiratory failure. It is important for you to remember that finding it difficult to breath, for whatever reason is a frightening experience and that these animals must not be stressed further by placing in a noisy and busy environment.

- Establish and maintain an airway

- Provide oxygen if necessary (refer to Chapter 40)
- Avoid stress and excessive handling of the patient
- Closely observe the respiratory pattern, noting changes in depth and character of the breaths
- Administer appropriate medications carefully by mouth
- Provide assisted feeding if necessary, these patients are often inappetent, but do not over stress by hand feeding

SEIZURES

Most seizures result in unconsciousness but are for a short duration of time, however, status epilepticus refers to continuous seizure activity and is classed as an emergency situation (refer to Chapter 42).

- Hospitalise the patient in a quiet stress-free environment with minimal stimulation
- If possible, darken the room and partially cover the front of the kennel door with a blanket, but ensure that observation of the patient is still possible
- Place an intravenous catheter to ensure easy vascular access in the event of a seizure
- Prepare antiseizure medication (usually diazepam) for rapid administration
- Do not try to restrain the patient during a convulsion
- Monitor, time and detail any seizure activity
- Maintain supportive treatment such as fluids and collect blood and urine samples as required for diagnostic and monitoring purposes

VOMITING ANIMALS

There are many things that cause the patient to vomit and treatment varies depending on the specific cause. However, the aim of therapy apart from removing the initiating cause is to control the vomiting episodes and avoid associated complications such as dehydration, electrolyte and acid-base imbalances and abdominal pain. It is important to remember that clinical signs of dehydration are not evident until the animal is quite significantly dehydrated.

- Observe for signs of nausea and administer anti-emetic as prescribed by the veterinary surgeon

APPENDICES

- Observe the patient for signs of dehydration
- Observe and record contents of vomit
- Offer small amounts of water or electrolyte solutions, but do not leave bowl in kennel
- Handle gently, abdominal area may be very painful
- Syringe fluids carefully to avoid aspiration pneumonia
- Clear vomitus away from animal's fur and kennel as soon as it is expelled
- Withhold food for 12 hours
- Assess hydration status and initiate intravenous fluid therapy if necessary

If and when the vomiting has ceased, small amounts of bland food such as fish, chicken or appropriate prescription diet may be given three to four times a day. Initially, give only a quarter of the daily allowance, and increase gradually over the following days until normal feeding amounts and food can be given.

CARE PLANS FOR PATIENTS POSTOPERATIVELY

Following surgery, the patient is returned to the ward area and the veterinary nurse must provide after-care aimed at preventing potential postoperative complications resulting from either the surgery or anaesthetic. More information with regard to postanaesthetic care is given in Chapter 22 with specific regard to management of hypothermia and analgesia. The following care plans are designed to highlight potential problems and specific nursing care relating to common surgical procedures.

Respiratory and circulatory complications and fluid and electrolyte imbalances are potential problems following any surgical procedure and you should be able to recognise them and act appropriately. More details are given in Chapters 40 and 41.

POSTOPERATIVE WOUNDS

Surgical wounds do not usually show evidence of infection (redness, swelling exudate, etc.) immediately following surgery. However, the wound is most susceptible to contamination in the initial postoperative period. Usually the patient is hospitalised during this period and so general ward and personal hygiene is essential to help prevent postoperative wound infection.

- Wash hands and wear sterile gloves before examining the wound or changing the dressing
- Protect the wound from external contamination with a suitable dressing material (refer to Chapter 6) for the first 48 hours
- Observe for evidence of haemorrhage at the wound site
- Prevent licking/interference by applying appropriate bandage or Elizabethan collar
- Reapply appropriate dressing material at recommended periods to enhance wound healing

ABDOMINAL SURGERY

A serious complication of abdominal surgery is secondary peritonitis, which can lead to serious systemic illness and unless treated aggressively can be fatal. The onset of peritonitis is usually acute, occurring several hours to a few days following the surgery. Clinical signs include pyrexia (although if already shocked, the patient may be hypothermic), tachycardia, dehydration, abdominal pain and signs associated with hypodynamic septic shock. Close monitoring of the patient is essential in the initial postoperative period so early detection and treatment can provide the best possible prognosis.

- Observe the patient for signs of nausea, vomiting and abdominal pain
- Maintain intravenous fluid therapy until the patient is able to meet its fluid requirements orally
- Offer small amounts of water by mouth after the anaesthetic recovery, carefully observing the patient
- After the initial food/water withholding time, encourage the patient to eat and drink to aid a return to normal gut peristalsis and electrolyte and nutrient assimilation.
- Gradually return to the patient's normal diet and feeding quantities over the following few days

AURAL SURGERY

The most frequently performed surgery to the ear includes drainage of aural haematomas, lateral wall resections and ear canal ablations. Following most aural surgery, the pinna of the affected ear is bandaged over the head to prevent excessive movements and head shaking (refer to Chapter 6). Facial nerve paralysis is a complication following canal surgery and may cause drooping of the eyelids and lips and dysphagia. These injuries usually resolve within a number of weeks, but the patient may require additional nursing care in the meantime.

- Check the head bandage frequently to ensure that it has not slipped or become too tight
- Change bandages and dressing every 1–3 days
- Clean the wound area gently using a mild povidone-iodine solution to remove crusts, discharge and haemorrhage
- Protect wound and bandage from self-trauma using an Elizabethan collar
- Observe the patient for evidence of facial nerve paralysis and apply an eye lubricant if required and as prescribed by the veterinary surgeon
- Observe patient eating and assist if necessary

CRYOSURGERY

The postoperative changes that occur in the cryosurgical patient are quite profound and can distress an unprepared owner. The whole point of cryosurgery is to destroy tissues by freezing. This of course results in tissue necrosis and sloughing which is most often the most disturbing aspect of cryosurgery visually. The frozen tissues undergo necrosis and a scab forms to protect the underlying healing tissues. This usually sloughs off in about 10 days to reveal a granulating wound.

- Apply a dressing and if possible, a pressure bandage over the area. Swelling and haemorrhage are common within hours of treatment but should resolve within 48 hours.
- Clean the area daily with a mild povidone-iodine solution. If freezing involves mucous membranes or if the patient interferes with the site, the scab becomes moist and may smell offensive.
- Prevent self-trauma by fitting an Elizabethan collar.
- If the animal becomes anorexic, hand feed highly palatable food.

GASTRIC DILATION

Gastric dilatation-volvulus-torsion is a medical and surgical emergency and the immediate first aid measures have been discussed in Chapter 42. Potential complications in the patient recovering postoperatively from surgery to correct the condition include hypovolaemic shock, septic-endotoxic shock, arrhythmias and abdominal pain. Close observation is essential to detect any such complications early and prevent the situation becoming life threatening.

- Check core body temperature and treat hypothermia.
- Maintain fluid and electrolyte balance and ensure appropriate fluids are being administered at the suitable rate. (Rates of up to 90 ml/kg/hour may be required during the initial therapy period.)
- Observe for cardiac arrhythmias using electrocardiogram (ECG).
- Measure and record packed cell volume (PCV), sodium and potassium levels frequently (hypokalaemia is the most common electrolyte imbalance).
- Monitor urine output.
- Withhold oral food and water for 24 hours postoperatively.
- Start feeding after this period with small amounts of bland, liquidised food and watch patient following feeding for regurgitation.
- Raise the food bowl to help prevent aerophagia.

GASTROINTESTINAL SURGERY

Surgery to the gastrointestinal tract is a fairly commonly performed procedure in small animal practice, frequently for the removal of a foreign body. Postoperatively, leakage from the gastric or intestinal incision can occur and peritonitis result. You must be fully aware of the clinical signs of septic shock so that identification can be picked up early and treatment instigated. In addition to the nursing care identified in the Abdominal Surgery Care Plan the following should be done:

- Observe the patient for evidence of septic shock for the entire hospitalisation period
- Offer small amounts of water after the anaesthetic recovery

- If water is retained, small quantities of food may be offered 12–24 hours following surgery. Food should be bland, for example, rice, boiled chicken or fish

OPHTHALMIC SURGERY

Depending on the surgery involved it may be necessary to administer a number of different topical eye treatments. It is important that at least 5 minutes are left between administration of the different drops to allow absorption. Ophthalmic procedures range from eyelid surgery to intraocular surgery but general principles include:

- Fit an Elizabethan collar *before* the patient recovers from the anaesthetic as eye surgery can be painful and these animals will often rub their eyes with their paws during the anaesthetic recovery period.
- Approach visually impaired animals slowly and talk to them gently so as not to startle them.
- Carry blind or poorly sighted animals outside rather than taking on the lead, but if they are too heavy, lead them around obstacles and keep the leash short so they remain close to your side.
- Make up eye drop administration chart if topical applications are being administered frequently and record all treatment times.
- Carefully clean away discharges and crusts from around the eye using moistened cotton wool balls with eyewash or other suitable isotonic solution. Avoid touching or rubbing the eyeball itself.
- Following intraocular surgery, position the patient with the head higher than the body during the recovery period to help reduce the risk of retinal separation.

ORAL/DENTAL SURGERY

Surgery to the oral cavity includes repair of lacerated tongue, tumour removal, salivary mucocele, maxilla/mandible – ectomy and tooth extraction. After any oral procedure, there is a risk of inhalation of blood and/or mucous and you should check for airway obstruction frequently.

- Ensure that gauze sponges and mouth packs have been removed from the pharynx
- Open mouth periodically to check for haemorrhage
- Keep mouth clear of blood and saliva using swabs or suction
- Observe patient closely for evidence of coughing or choking
- Raise the patient's body and lower their head so that fluids drain out of the mouth
- Offer water when the patient has regained consciousness but withhold food for the first 24 hours
- After 24 hours, provide soft, moist food and hand feed if necessary
- If the animal tries to scratch its face, fit an Elizabethan collar or bandage the feet if the collar interferes with the surgical area

ORTHOPAEDIC SURGERY

Osteomyelitis is one of the most serious risks associated with orthopaedic surgery and therefore it is essential that you pay close attention to and record vital signs. The veterinary surgeon must be informed of any pain, swelling or discharging sinuses so that immediate action in the form of radiographs, bacteriology and sensitivity analysis and introduction of antibiotics can be initiated.

- Immediately following surgery, obtain core body temperature and treat hypothermia.
- Observe patient closely for signs of pain and inform VS as necessary.
- Keep the surgical wound clean and apply sterile dressing over incisional wound. Check, clean and change dressing daily.
- Ensure that all dressings and bandages are kept clean and dry and examine frequently to ensure that circulation is not compromised.
- Cover limb bandages and casts when taking the animal outside for exercise with a protective covering. An empty fluid bag with the bottom cut off makes a useful and tough cover. Always remove covering as soon as the animal is returned to the kennel.
- Support and assist patients with multiple fractures during exercise using a towel sling.
- Fit an Elizabethan collar if the patient interferes with the bandage or cast.

- Initiate physiotherapy if indicated but do not perform treatment over newly repaired fracture site.
- Consider high protein diet following surgery and high calorie requirement of patient.

OVARIOHYSTERECTOMY/PYOMETRA

Ovariohysterectomy is one of the most commonly performed surgical procedures in many small animal clinics. With such a routine procedure it is easy to become blasé about the postoperative care of these animals and provide inadequate monitoring of the animal. You should remember, however, that haemorrhage is the most common cause of death following this type of surgery. Following ovariohysterectomy for pyometra, there is the additional complication of septic shock and you must be fully familiar with the associated clinical signs.

In addition to the complications and nursing care given to any patient following abdominal surgery:

- Monitor the patient closely for evidence of haemorrhage and hypovolaemic shock. (Check for haemorrhage from the abdominal incision, abdominal swelling, pale mucous membranes, depression and weak, rapid pulse.)
- Monitor closely for evidence of septic shock, which includes the typical signs of hypovolaemic shock such as tachycardia, tachypnoea, but instead the patient may show an elevated core body temperature and brick-red mucous membranes.

SPINAL SURGERY

These patients require intensive nursing care. Spinal surgery can take several hours and hypothermia is common postoperatively as a result.

- Immediately following surgery, obtain core temperature and treat hypothermia as necessary. Remember that these animals may be physically unable to move away from heat sources so ensure burns do not occur from heat pads or lamps.
- Closely observe the patient for evidence of pain and refer to VS (opioids are most commonly used for the first 24 hours).
- Confine the animal to a small area to prevent too much movement.

- Provide lots of padding such as water beds, thick foam mattresses and 'Vetbed' style bedding.
- Prevent skin contact with urine and faeces by using a non-retentive bedding material such as 'Vetbed'. Application of white soft paraffin is also useful.
- Note the patient's ability to urinate and defecate and manually express or catheterise the bladder to prevent overflow or urine retention.
- Check the incisional area for evidence of swelling or haemorrhage.
- Apply ice pack and pressure wraps if necessary.
- Turn the patient 4-hourly to help prevent hypostatic pneumonia.
- Prevent decubital ulcers by protecting bony prominences.
- Perform a neurological examination daily.
- Provide physiotherapy three to four times daily to maintain muscle tone.
- Assist paraplegic dogs to walk using slings or a towel under the abdomen.

THORACIC SURGERY

As with all lengthy surgical procedures, hypothermia is extremely common postoperatively. In this case, a return to normal body temperature is particularly important because hypothermia and shivering increase oxygen consumption and decrease ventilatory capacity.

- Provide a quiet, stress-free environment so as not to aggravate existing respiratory insufficiency
- During recovery, place patient in lateral recumbency with the side of the thoracotomy uppermost (if lateral thoracotomy incision performed)
- Observe the patient closely for signs of respiratory distress and evidence of postoperative pain (pain from a thoracotomy wound may prevent normal respiratory excursions and worsen ventilatory efforts)
- If available, measure tidal volume (should be no less than 10 ml/kg) using a Wright's respirometer and check oxygenation with a pulse oximeter
- Thoracic bandages help seal the thoracotomy wound and reduce emphysema around the incision, but it is imperative that it is not too tight and restricting ventilation

APPENDICES

- Position patient on to sternal recumbency as soon as possible to allow both lungs to expand and minimise congestion
- Check thoracic drains frequently and record quantities of fluid/haemorrhage/air present in the chest bottle
- Ensure drainage bottles are placed and maintained at least 1 metre below the patient providing a suction pressure of 5–10 cm of water
- Remove drainage tubes as soon as possible, as a general guide, the tube can be removed if less than 100 ml of fluid is being drawn off over a 24-hour period
- Provide supplementary oxygen therapy if necessary

URINARY TRACT

Surgery includes nephrectomy, ureteric ectopia correction, cystotomy and urethrostomy. Following surgery to the urinary tract, temporary urinary obstruction may occur due to swelling postoperatively.

- Monitor urine output. Measure accurately if an indwelling catheter is placed or estimate the quantity if not.
- Observe patient closely for evidence of tenesmus, haematuria and pain on urination.
- Prevent urine scalding from overflow or leakage by applying a barrier cream such as white soft paraffin.
- Prevent self-trauma by fitting an Elizabethan collar.
- Maintain urinary catheters and collection bag systems. (Refer to care plans for general conditions).
- Provide plenty of opportunities for the patient to urinate by taking outside frequently or providing a clean litter tray.

FURTHER READING

Darke, P.G.G. (1986) *Notes on Canine Internal Medicine,* 2nd edn. Wright Imprint, Bristol, UK.

Houlton, J.E.F. & Taylor P.M. (1987) *Trauma Management in the Dog and Cat.* Wright Imprint, Bristol, UK

Taylor R. & McGehee R. (1995) *Manual of Small Animal Postoperative Care.* Lea & Fabiger, Philadelphia, USA.

APPENDIX 2

CALCULATIONS

For

- Percentages of solutions
- Anaesthetic gas flow rates
- Fluid therapy rates
- Calorie requirements
- Radiography calculations

CALCULATING SOLUTIONS AND DRUG DOSE RATES

% solution = (weight (g) × 100) ÷ volume of solution (ml)

volume of solution (ml) = (weight (g) × 100) ÷ % solution

weight (g) = (volume of solution (ml) × % solution) ÷ 100

Remember that:

- 1 ml of solution weighs 1 g
- 1 g = 1000 mg
- A 1% solution contains 1 g in 100 ml
- A 2% solution contains 2 g in 100 ml, and so on
- A 10% solution contains 10 mg/ml

If you know that an animal needs a certain amount of mg of a drug, but do not know how many ml or tablets that is, you can use this formula to work it out:

dose prescribed (mg)/dose per ml or concentration

Example

A dog needs 25 mg of a drug to be given by injection, and the drug is in a strength of 50 mg/ml:

25 mg ÷ 50 mg = 0.5 ml

CALCULATING ANAESTHETIC GAS FLOW RATES

Tidal volume = the amount of gas passing into and out of the lungs in one breath. This is estimated at 10–15 ml/kg.

Minute volume = the volume of air inhaled or exhaled in one minute.

FORMULA FOR WORKING OUT FLOW RATE

The animal's tidal volume must be calculated first:
- Tidal volume = 10–15 ml/kg
- Cats/small dogs = 15 ml/kg
- Medium/large dogs = 10 ml/kg

To find out the minute volume, multiply the tidal volume by the respiration rate per minute.

Then multiply this by the circuit factor:

- Ayres T-Piece & Bain = 2.5–3
- Magill & Lack = 1–1.5

The whole formula is:

body weight × 10–15 × respiration rate × circuit factor

Example

What would the flow rate be for a 30 kg dog with a respiration rate of 20/min?

30 (body weight) × 10 (tidal volume) × 20 (respiration rate) × 1.5 (circuit factor) = 9000 ml (9 litres)

CALCULATING FLUID THERAPY DRIP RATES

The maintenance fluid requirement is the amount of fluid normally required by the patient over a certain period. This is calculated at approximately 50 ml/kg/24 hours

WORKING OUT THE NUMBER OF DROPS PER SECOND

The drip rate must be worked out. Different giving sets administer different amounts of drops per ml.

- Paediatric giving set = 60 drops/ml
- General giving sets = 20 drops/ml

So, the amount required:

Total amount in 24 hours ÷ 24 = hourly rate

hourly rate ÷ 60 = minute rate

minute rate × giving set drip factor = number of drops per min

60 ÷ drops per min = the second rate

Example
A 15 kg dog needs 750 ml over 24 hours. A giving set is used that delivers 20 drops/ml.

750 ÷ 24 = 31.25

31.25 ÷ 60 = 0.52

0.52 × 20 = 10.4

60 ÷ 10.4 = 5.7

So the giving set should be set at one drop approximately every 6 seconds.

CALCULATING CALORIE REQUIREMENTS

Basal energy requirement (BER) for dogs over 5 kg = 30 × (body weight kg) + 70

BER for small dogs and cats under 5 kg = 60 × (body weight kg)

Then multiply by the 'disease factor':

Cage rest	1.2
Surgery/trauma	1.3
Multiple surgery/trauma	1.5
Sepsis/neoplasia	1.7
Burns	2.0
Growth	2.0

This total figure = the amount of Kcal required over 24 hours.
Example
A 25 kg dog following surgery would require:

$(30 \times 25 + 70) \times 1.3 = 1066$ Kcal/day

CALCULATING RADIOGRAPHIC EXPOSURES

FILM FOCAL DISTANCE AND THE INVERSE SQUARE LAW

If you alter the FFD, the new exposure can be worked out using this calculation:

new mAs = new FFD^2 ÷ old FFD^2 × old mAs

Example
Having been using an exposure of 10 mAs and FFD of 50 cm, what exposure is required if the FFD is changed to 100 cm?

Answer: $10 \times 10\,000 \div 2500 = 40$ mAs.

THE 10 kV RULE

- Increase the kV by 10 and you can halve the mAs.
- Decrease the kV by 10 and you can double the mAs.

If you need to keep the actual image the same, but need to alter the exposure, the 10 kV rule works like this:
50 kV at 32 mAs will create the same exposure as:
60 kV at 16 mAs and
70 kV at 8 mAs
So, if an exposure at 20 mAs at 80 kV is adequate, what is the kV required if the mAs are changed to 10?
Answer: The mAs are halved therefore increase kV by 10 = 90 kV.

MILLIAMPERAGE (mA) AND TIME (s)

$$mAs = mA \times s$$

If mA is doubled, the time may be halved (thereby decreasing exposure time and reducing the possibility of movement blur).

GRID FACTOR

$$mAs \times grid\ factor\ (GF) = exposure\ required\ using\ grid$$

For example: the exposure factors required for a lateral radiograph of a dog's abdomen might be 3.2 mAs at 80 kV.
If a grid with a grid factor of 3 is used, the new exposure will be:

$$3.2 \times 3 = 9.6\ mAs\ at\ 80\ kV.$$

This may be rather too much time and so the 10 kV rule can be used. By increasing the kV by 10 it is possible to halve the mAs, giving a setting of 90 kV at 4.8 mAs.

INDEX

INDEX

INDEX